If you wish to know
how many friends
you have,
buy
a
cottage on a lake.

If you should wish your
summer to be short,
borrow some
money and
have it
due
in
the fall.

If you wish to lose
weight, never eat
more than you
can lift.

THE
FABULOUS
SEX ORGAN
DIET

JOHN VAN REGINALD TOMLINSON III
DIETARY SCIENTIST

THE BEAVER ISLAND TRADING COMPANY
Founded 1983

FABULOUS SEX ORGAN DIET

Edited by
David Kinder
Amanda Winnicki

Cartoons
Bill Toll

Printed in the United States of America
First printing ... April 1991
Second printing ... June 1991
Third printing... September 1991

ISBN: 0-9629805-0-1

Library of Congress
Catalog Card Number 91-072614

For information address: Beaver Island Trading Co.
P.O. Box 157
Flint, Michigan 48501

Contents

Dedicated to my dear darling wife
Lori, who went on this diet
and lost so much weight
I had to start feeding her
milkshakes so she
didn't waste away
to nothing.

CAVEAT EMPTOR

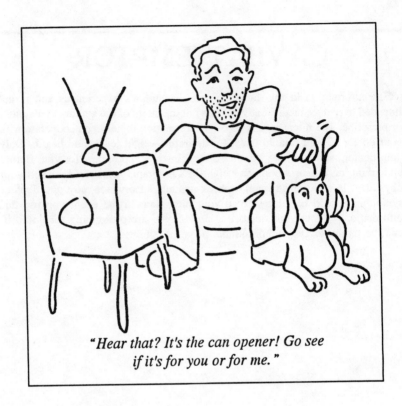

"Hear that? It's the can opener! Go see
if it's for you or for me."

Introduction -
A NEW BEGINNING

I was talking to a friend of mine the other day and he said, "You know, if I knew I was going to live this long, I would have taken better care of myself." The guy's forty two. His name - Jim Moshenko. He desperately wants to do something about his physique but isn't sure what. He's considering exercise, but only because it's been so long since he's heard any heavy breathing, he misses it (the heavy breathing). He has no idea what THE FABULOUS SEX ORGAN DIET can do for him, but he saw what it did for me. That's why the last time he saw me he said, "Fax me the details and we'll do lunch." Yeah, right.

But after I determined that his interest in seeing this extravaganza in print was real, I took the journal I kept while doing crazed dietary experiments on myself, and used it as the basis for a more comprehensive work (you'll find the journal, which is chapter 7, exciting reading). My degree in science has given me the skill to perform the kind of in depth research necessary to lend credibility to the ideas I've spawned, and no matter how outrageous they may appear at first glance, they work! As a result, I can honestly say, based on everything I've learned from my research, that you've embarked on a journey that's sure to change your life forever. If you never were a special person before, you're a special person now! Further, if you doubt what I'm saying, you're probably hallucinating.

The most important concept behind this book, as far as I'm concerned, is that the diet conforms to the American way of doing things. Which, in essence means that it's easy, great fun, and of course, quick and simple. There can be absolutely no pain or strain in the All American Diet, and the results must certainly be immediate. Is there any doubt in your mind that we, as Americans, have the God given right to the best of diets? With this in mind, I'm pleased to announce that THE FABULOUS SEX ORGAN DIET will fulfill your every dietary desire. Of this you can be sure. THE FABULOUS SEX ORGAN DIET will not leave you frustrated at the end of the night, feeling like you should have gotten more than you did.

Another thrust of this book, is to make you laugh out loud. Due to the fact that there seems to be very little dietary laughter around, many of us have instead been forced to laugh at our sex life. Let's face it, if food wasn't any more plentiful than sex, we'd all be trying to figure out how to gain weight, instead of trying to lose it. Studies seem to indicate that people fantasize a great deal more about food than even about sex. It's probably because at least when you're done fantasizing about food, you can go get some.

You may love to eat and love to have sex, but in terms of the frequency of repetition, eating's going to win out just about every day. You may think I'm kidding, but believe me, it's a lot easier to eat three meals a day. The interesting thing about this is due to the fact that we do get so many more chances to eat than to have sex, it's possible to eat all the time, and yet go so long without sex that you can't even remember who gets tied up!

That's why diet books outsell sex books three to one. If you're going to improve, you might as well improve at something you do all the time, especially if the improvement will leave you permanently better as a human being. That's why the thrust of this book is clearly about losing weight and more importantly, about laughing at our past. As a first step, I think it's important to remember that we need to lighten up mentally <u>before</u> we can lighten up physically. Bearing down on yourself isn't going to do it. You might just be heavy because you've got the whole world on your shoulders and you're eating to find the strength to bear up under the strain. Believe me, having the whole world on your shoulders can make you feel like you weigh a ton!

Furthermore, in so many of the books and scientific journals I've studied while doing the research for this magnum opus of mine, I've been forcibly struck by the inescapable fact that the science of diet and nutrition can be terminally dull. This is, as far as I'm concerned, a major flaw in any book trying to inspire you to take action to deal with the problem. So don't hesitate to lighten up mentally first, and laugh uproariously, should the urge possess you.

I would further urge you to forego thinking of this as another quick-fix diet that may enable you to lose a great deal of weight quickly, but as luck would have it, you end up finding it again, just as quickly, once you stop jumping through the recommended dietary hoops. I want you to begin to consider the possibility that it's time to go to a new level and become permanently better, rather than slamming your ham around on the now infamous diet roller coaster.

I've talked to professional dieters who've lost literally thousands of pounds in their lifetime, and yet they're still overweight today. Are you one of these professional dieters? Fortunately, if you are, you will soon see that this isn't the kind of diet that requires you to be a strict disciplinarian, unless of course you're strictly an octogenarian, in which case, speed is most certainly everything. Actually, if you're over eighty, you might think about dropping this diet idea and consider a junk food diet simply because you probably need all the preservatives you can get!

One thing you'll find right away is that the more you apply the principles outlined in this book, the better you'll feel. The more you let this feeling of well being grow inside you, the more you're going to get excited about becoming permanently better. Health does that to a person! Before you know it, the new will be replacing the old at such an incredible rate that you'll be ordering multiple copies of this famous work for friends who probably need it even more than you do. If that's the case, you'd better order now, while you can still get the free bonus!

Which brings me to the reason you bought the book in the first place. I'm going to go out on a limb and guess that it was for one of the following reasons: 1) you've never heard of anything so patently outrageous and wanted to find out what it was all about; 2) you're really interested in losing weight and are willing to try almost anything; 3) you really enjoy fine literature; 4) you're thinking of having kids and are wondering if this will be an aid to fertilization; and 5) you just want to get laid and will try anything.

If any, or all of the above reasons inspired you to purchase this, you're in luck! When you finally come to realize the full ramifications of the truly exciting information contained herein, you will be so personally excited by the prospect of a new life without the pitfalls that even the biggest dieters sometimes succumb to, that you'll drop the idea of suicide.

Here's something to contemplate: Is it impossible for an optimist to be pleasantly surprised?

Everybody in the world seems amazed at just what Americans are willing to eat. The ironic thing about it is that when you consider how indifferent Americans are to the quality and cooking of the food they put into their mouths, it can only strike you as peculiar, that they should take such pride in the mechanical devices they use for its excretion. I mention this because help is where you find it, and this little fascination, as you'll soon discover during the course of your reading, can be turned to your distinct advantage. Fore, even though modern technology has adequately dealt with where the food goes once we're finally rid of it, it's the stuff that's staying behind that's doing the damage. So we're going to learn how to take this little miracle of man and improve our process of elimination to accelerate weight loss.

Question; If there were a way to give yourself a five minute motor flush every day with breakfast, one that would make the process of elimination more effective when it comes to eliminating the material responsible for your weight problem, would you be interested?

John Lennon, God rest his soul, said it best when he so poignantly pronounced that we are what we eat. The obvious meaning to this statement, as you have almost certainly deduced, is that what is eaten today is employed in the manufacture of cells in the body tomorrow. Scientists maintain that the body is completely rebuilt cell by cell every five to seven years. If this is indeed true, and if it is also true that for many Americans, their dietary regimen has led them to become something of a cross between a compost and a compactor, then I have another question for you.

Do you really want to be tomorrow what you've eaten today?

In order to dispel a common misconception about diets, I would like to add a note of clarification at this point. Somehow we've gotten the idea that a diet is some special program relating to the consumption of foodstuffs that one embarks upon when one desires to lose weight. Nothing could be further from the truth. Unless you have given up eating altogether, in which case you will be with us only a short while longer, you are always on some sort of diet. It may or may not be organized and it certainly might not be recommended by leading authorities in the field of oral intake (even though they may be interested in studying you later at some point to determine just what the digestive tract is capable of), but it is a diet! So what you're going to do with THE FABULOUS SEX ORGAN DIET is to alter your diet just a little, to tweak it if you will. This will allow you to receive the maximum benefit from that which you eat, whatever that may be.

Question; If no matter what you eat, you're on a diet of some sort, can you adjust your thinking to allow you to start thinking in terms of refueling, revitalizing, cleansing and re-energizing your body with the fuel of the Patriot, rather than the fuel of the Scud?

In essence, we here at THE FABULOUS SEX ORGAN DIET CO. are counting on the fact that you will be what you eat. The key for me will be to show you with words, pictures, and emotions, just how eating raw sex organs will fill you with the life giving energy you were always meant to have from the beginning, and make you permanently better!

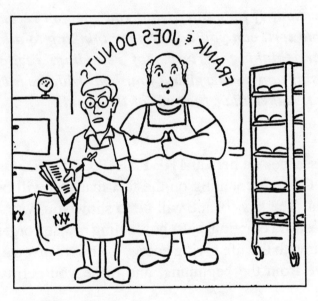

*"Well, shoot. I just can't figure it out. I'm
movin' over 500 doughnuts a day, but
I'm still just barely squeakin' by."*

Chapter 1 -
THE BEAUTY OF THE BODY

The miracle of the body is more to the point! One of the greatest miracles of all time still cannot be explained by the scientific community. What is this miracle? It is simply that nobody, at least nobody in the scientific community, can tell you, or me for that matter, what is the motive force that propels us and keeps us "living." Sure, they can tell you what will happen if organs fail to function or if the ongoing processes of the body are interrupted. But there is absolutely no scientific ability to either identify or quantify the LIFEFORCE within us.

In fact, I believe that the bulk of the scientists now studying the body would agree that there is so much more that we don't know than what we do know, that there is literally no comparison! The point is that while there is plenty of speculation on what drives us, it is still one of the cosmic unknowns in science. In fact, there is a vast amount within the scientific realm that scientists can't seem to agree on. As an example, psychology is an area where scientific thinking is all over the map. Psychologists regularly accuse each other of being crazy! The field of nutrition is another. While most nutritionists can agree on the basic food groups, they don't agree on much else.

That's why THE FABULOUS SEX ORGAN DIET is so cosmic. There is nothing to disagree with, because it allows you to bring your natural bodily processes into harmony, naturally. There is no quackery or pseudoscience in the diet. It simply organizes what is now known into a way of living that makes you feel wonderful! If you've been living with your body for more than twenty years, you know it fairly well. The fact that it can keep going in spite of all you've done to it, is testament to what a miracle it really is. So let's look at this miracle that keeps us going.

As a machine it's unparalleled. There is no technology being developed on this planet that even approximates the ability of the body as a continuously operating, updating, continually reproducing, and extremely mobile machine. We don't have to talk about critical organs such as the brain, heart, lungs, skin, liver, or the reproductive system, when looking for miracles, just look at the hand, or even the thumb: the smartest people in the world can't even begin to make a mechanism as versatile as the thumb.

We can build machinery to put a man on the moon, but even simple functions involving THE LIFEFORCE cannot be replicated in the laboratory. You were constructed with equipment that was incredibly well designed and constantly services itself. (I have to service myself all the time and it still amazes me what a wonderful thing it is.) The point is that even with the vast store of accumulated knowledge mankind has at it's fingertips, it cannot make anything like your body!

Let me tell you about your equipment... Let's take the red blood cell as one microscopic example. It's a tiny, round disc that drops off carbon dioxide, and picks up oxygen as it passes quickly through the lungs. It drops off the oxygen at the doorstep of a cell somewhere in the body, and then picks up the carbon dioxide, which is a waste product of cellular combustion, and takes it back to the lung to begin the cycle anew. In the six quarts of blood you have in your system, there are twenty-four trillion of these little suckers. In fact, your body makes about seven million of these little diskettes every second. Your body even creates white blood cells to come along and clean up the mess when they break apart and die. White blood cells are like a janitorial service, so everything stays nice and clean throughout the system.

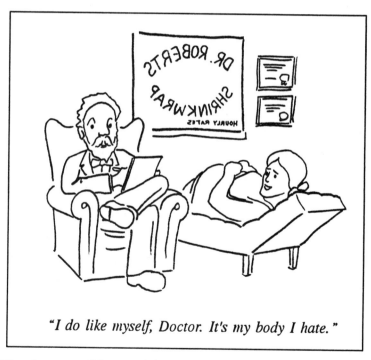

"I do like myself, Doctor. It's my body I hate."

Here's something I think is kind of cosmic. Since the function of these blood cells is observable, a group of scientists got together and decided to use a complex computer analysis program to design the perfect shape for a red blood cell, considering all it does. The shape must permit unencumbered flow in a closed system and yet have tremendous absorption capabilities so that no inefficiency occurs. Inefficiency would be an area within the shape that isn't able to absorb oxygen, as the cell passes through the lung. This inefficiency would create an empty area within the cell shape causing wasted effort.

Guess what! After everything was fed into the computer, considering every known geometric shape, the perfect design turned out to be the exact shape of the red blood cell.

That's only the beginning. Consider the fact that the heart has to beat about one hundred thousand times every twenty four hours, and can do this decade after decade without so much as a missed beat, unless of course you sneeze. It pumps six quarts of liquid through a system of arteries, veins, and capillaries, that if stuck together as one long tube, would stretch around the equator of the earth four times. That's a long way to pump anything! But the truly remarkable thing about the heart is that, for all the beating it does, it rests far more than it works. That's why it doesn't get tired for eighty or ninety years!

The intelligence inherent in our system is so immense, that it is incomprehensible to even the most insightful of geniuses who ever lived. Any system that can keep almost one hundred trillion cells (In terms of numbers, this is literally thousands of times the current population of the earth.) functioning in perfect harmony, is very good! As you are already familiar with the difficulty coordinating the activities of just the four billion or so people we have here on earth, imagine the difficulty of controlling many times that number and doing it smoothly in an environment completely hostile to human life. If it weren't for built in self preservation systems like the immune system, germs alone would kill us shortly after birth, if we made it that far. Further, it not only has numerous systems and sensors built in to keep it on track, it has systems built in to get it back on track, should it somehow derail!

There is the endocrine system which produces hormones for everything from stimulating various body functions to protecting us from perceived dangers, both in and out of the body. There is the temperature control mechanism, with its four million pores, that controls everything from sweating, to expanding or contracting the blood vessels, depending upon whether the body is trying to conserve or eliminate the heat. The system will constrict vessels and give you goose bumps if they're needed (which by the way will increase surface metabolism up to 400%) in order to keep the body at 98.6 degrees Fahrenheit, and you don't even have to think about it.

There's the dream mechanism that enables the brain to release destructive stress and solve problems. Did you know that if you completely stopped dreaming you would go insane in several weeks, and that studies done by the University of Chicago among others have clearly demonstrated the ability to induce insanity in humans by preventing the mind from dreaming. The interesting thing about how this protection mechanism works is that, in the study, once dreaming was allowed to recommence, the mind made up all the dreaming time for which it was deprived, until all the lost time was made up. Additionally, just as the symptoms of mental illness increased in severity as dream time was lost, as dream time was made up by the brain, the symptoms recessed in the reverse order that they appeared. Finally when all the dream time was made up, the symptoms disappeared completely.

Another of the many miracles that keep us alive, is the miracle of the five senses. Then there is; the ingenious system of semi-circular canals in the inner ear to provide balance; the 25 billion cells that make up the brain, most of which we still haven't learned to use, and of course the lymph system, that even I don't fully understand! We have a reproductive system that absolutely defies laboratory duplication of even the smallest part. We have a well developed system for regularly feeding and otherwise nourishing almost one hundred trillion cells every single day. Can you imagine even keeping track of what that many different cells want every day?

While we're at it, let's look at one of these cells. Even though they're too small to see with the nude eye, individual cells are millions of times larger than their smallest components. A cell carries on, in little organelles, every function that is found in the body as a whole. There's even a little "brain" in there. It also stores and burns energy, just like the body. It takes in food and eliminates waste. It likes to party and carry on, and even has sex with itself. I wonder if they ever say, "Gee, I've got a headache, I really don't feel like dividing tonight?"

When you put it all together, you've got a big miracle on your hands. You've got a brain that has to not only oversee the care and feeding of all those cells (while the cells work feverishly to follow the brain's commands), but must execute trillions of different intricate processes on an on-going basis. When you think about all the things the body must do, simply to stay alive, and then you throw in all the things that you personally have planned (like go to work and make some money to pay for the good time you showed those cells last weekend), you've got to admit, the body has its work cut out for it!

Meanwhile, it's keeping you breathing seventy times a minute and following a preset growth plan encoded on a DNA string that is so small that all the DNA in every cell in your body will fit into something the size of an ice cube. Yet, if it were unwound, stretched out, and joined together, it would produce a string that would go from the earth to the sun and back over four hundred times. It works out to eighty billion miles of DNA. Now that's a hell of a lot of reading, but your cells have to read it regularly for guidance. After all that reading, it still has to have time to figure out what's for dinner.

In discussing just how amazingly intelligent your body is, the point I want to stress is, any body that can do all that yours does just to keep you alive, can figure out how much you're supposed to weigh. Wouldn't you agree? The work your body has to do minute by minute is clearly more than any of us could be hired to do, no matter what the wage. I know I'd hate to think of doing that much work.

So here's the question once again: Do you think a brain that can conduct literally quadrillions of different processes with pinpoint accuracy (at least 200 different reactions can be triggered in a single cell by a single enzyme, at any one point in time), a brain that can keep all things in harmony and balance, while fighting off a plethora of deadly germs, can figure out how much you're supposed to weigh and keep you at that weight?

Of course it can! Our genetic code has a complete plan

which outlines in great detail just what we should look like, and it doesn't include mounds of fat surrounding an otherwise perfect body. Your body is so smart that if you give it the opportunity, it will do whatever is necessary to bring you back to perfect health. All it needs is your cooperation. It doesn't mean starving yourself, or putting yourself through unnecessary hell in order to shed what your body already knows it doesn't need. It means getting in harmony with THE LIFEFORCE already within you. It means facilitating the process rather than thwarting it. In so doing, you and your body will be happy together, being serviced and getting serviced.

Who was it that said that a waist is a terrible thing to mind? Probably a dieter stuck with the arduous task of having to count calories. I'll bet you that most people haven't got the slightest idea what a calorie is. They only know it has to do with putting on or losing weight, which is only indirectly true. As an example, the furnace in your house burns tons of calories every day, yet it doesn't seem to get any smaller. It also takes in millions of calories every day, yet it doesn't get any bigger. How can that be?

The reason is that it doesn't store them as surplus bulk for future use. It takes in just what it needs to burn for heat to get the house up to a predesignated temperature, then it stops the intake. It's kind of like that business buzz word of the eighties, "just in time inventories." The idea is to keep the needed materials for construction down to just what is needed for the next day, and when that's "digested" the company gets more and the process continues.

A calorie is a measure of energy, heat energy to be exact. One calorie will raise one gram of water (this is a reasonably small amount of water) one degree Celsius or about one and three quarters of a degree Fahrenheit. So you can see that it actually takes quite a few of these to get any real work done. As an example, it takes a hundred of them just to boil a few drops of water, and when you think that your very own body is at least 70% water and must be kept at 98.6 degrees constantly, you can readily see that when you factor in your weight, your body has to burn literally thousands of calories every day even if you do nothing. One calorie in dietary terms is actually a kilo-calorie, or one thousand calories to a scientist. So when you burn approximately 2500 to 3500 dietary calories per day, depending on your sex and how active you are, you're burning one heck of a lot of fuel!

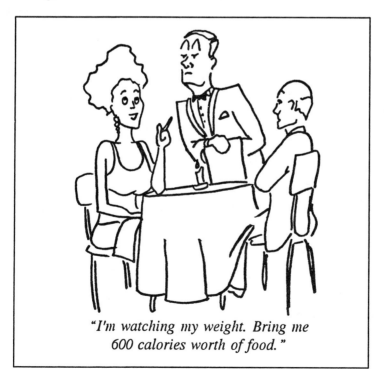

*"I'm watching my weight. Bring me
600 calories worth of food."*

So now you ask, "Fine, but what does all this have to do with my furnace and just in time inventories?" Well that's a good question and I'm glad you asked, because there are two similarities that I think are important to bring out. First, it's interesting to note that our bodies are no different in some respects from a manufacturing facility or a furnace, in that they both have an input which leads directly to an output.

They both have waste they must eliminate or get choked off, and the quality of the input directly affects the level and quality of the output. Poor quality steel means poor quality parts and increased scrap. This results in increased waste products that your company not only must waste valuable time disposing of, but your output is slowed while it does. Furthermore, it costs a company a great deal of money to get rid of this waste (in the case of your body, this means an expenditure of the free floating energy in the bloodstream). The quality of the output determines whether a company grows and thrives, or just languishes, barely getting by. Simply put, the output is determined by the input.

A furnace, although doing something completely different from your body, has to contend with the quality of the input. If the gas or oil is poorly refined, it will burn less efficiently, Therefore, the furnace becomes less productive and more expensive to operate. More importantly, waste in the form of soot begins to pile up on the burner, nozzles, and in the chimney. If not corrected, breakdowns will begin to occur as things get clogged, and parts must then be replaced. When the chimney gets plugged, the whole system backs up and things gets very messy. Thus creating more employment for the furnace "surgeons" and, at the same time, leaving you pissed off at the oil company for putting such poor quality fuel into your beautiful furnace.

Question; In a case like this, do you change oil companies or do you just keep paying to fix the damn thing?

The lesson here about minimizing waste to improve efficiency and controlling the quality of the input is vitally important whether we're talking about a manufacturing facility, a furnace, or your body. It's so important that it will be discussed quite a bit more in Chapter 5. But as I mentioned above, there are two similarities, and I would be remiss if I neglected to discuss the second similarity.

The second is potentially more important than the first. It concerns the body's control mechanism. Like the furnace, which has a thermostat to govern when fuel is burned to heat the regulated space, and the factory that uses a computer to monitor and control the extent to which inventories are needed for production, the body has a control mechanism governing the extent to which inventories are burned or accumulated for the conduction of internal affairs. In fact, your body can count calories much better than you can!

As you have no doubt already surmised, this all takes place in our own personal computer, the one just above the shoulders. This computer analogy is actually an old one. I'll bet you didn't know that computers were first talked about by Adam and Eve. That's right, as I recall the story, it was Eve that said to Adam, "I'll let you play with my Apple if I can play with your Wang."

Whether this first historical mention of the computer is factual or just another oral tradition is immaterial. The key for our purposes is to understand how to use the one in our head. We don't need to itemize its every function, or even to understand how it does what it does. All we need to know is how to set it (program it) and adjust it to do our bidding.

In this way it will help us accomplish our goals, rather than fight us every step of the way. Just imagine the uproar in any factory if inventory control didn't tell transportation, (which probably has a ton of stuff on the way), that the door will be closed to any new incoming inventories until further notice. It would be a mess. The same is true for our internal control system. Coordination between systems is essential!

All we really want is a brain that's user friendly. Just as we don't need to understand the inner workings of the thermostat in the hall to turn the heat up and down, we don't need to understand the inner workings of the brain to program it. You simply need to take the time to learn how the program works, and take a little time every day to play with it.

If you don't take the time to set your thermostat/ inventory control (TIC), your conscious mind, which determines your wants (as opposed to your needs, which are more a product of internal drives), will be doing battle with one of the strongest forces on earth: your subconscious mind. Unless you're one tough cookie (something like my grandma's molasses oatmeal supremes), you're going to have a tough time of it until either perseverance has indirectly reset your program, or your subconscious overwhelms your conscious mind and you fail to obtain what you want. Why do things the hard way? Relax and put your body on cruise! Here's how...

The language of the mind is made up of words, pictures and emotions stored as a reference guide. This is used in the analysis of all incoming data. The mind compares incoming data with what is previously stored, codifies it and files it, according to its importance and veracity. Sometimes the event responsible for the stored data is so dramatic, that it has a powerful effect on our lives from that point forward.

What happens is that powerful experiences have the same affect on our future actions as scratches on records. Just as a scratch blocks the needle's path and suddenly shifts it to a different groove (blocking the rest of that particular groove), new input into our mind is diverted by emotional scratches that can trigger emotional behavior that doesn't make sense to the uninitiated observer. The behavior is odd in the same way a song sounds odd to someone who's never heard it before and doesn't know about the scratch. That's why events like getting burned in love can have a chilling effect on future amorous adventures. Certainly the expression of needing to be "regrooved" is just as apt for behavior that shifts us away from our goals as it is for records with big scratches.

I call these scratches in our lives, DEFINING MO-MENTS, because they are so tremendously important to the way we act from that point forward. When our mind stores an idea with tremendous emotion attached, future incoming related data is sent right to the top of the importance list. There it gets filtered in a way that literally forces you to think in preconceived ways, like a scratch causes a skip. This will continue until you are able to finally (sometimes one never does) recolor the event or episode to better fit your current feeling on the matter.

In essence what this means, is that the stored words,

pictures, and emotions we carry in our data banks determine to a large extent, what we are and what we will become as individuals. Everyone has a TIC system that analyzes all incoming data in light of such factors as: feelings about ourself, how we view our strengths and weaknesses, and our ability to get things done.

The ironic thing about this ability of the mind is that the mind has absolutely no ability to distinguish between fact and fantasy. In other words, all the things you feel about yourself (which psychologists call the self image) are based rightly or wrongly, for better or for worse, for richer or poorer, in sickness and in health, on stored videos that could just as easily be a delusion as a real event. A prime example is the kid who is deathly afraid of spiders because of the monster spider he used to imagine as being under his bed and ready to eat him every night when he went to sleep. His fear is as real as if a monster spider were actually there.

The mind stores everything you feel at the same time that it's storing what you see, even if what you see is only in the mind. That's why when you think back you can remember how you felt when a past event comes to mind. Often we can re-experience these emotions all over again when viewing one of these videos, because they're right on the film with the sound. If you think back to a DEFINING MOMENT in your life (and I'm not necessarily talking about something sixty seconds long, DEFINING MO-MENTS can transpire over a period of several months), that led you to make a major change in either the way you do things or the way you are as a person, or maybe both, there was a powerful emotion tied to an idea, and from that point on, your life was a reaction to the strength of that emotional feeling.

This same concept, that of producing change by tying a strong emotion to an exciting idea, is at the very heart of a great motivational speaker's effectiveness. It's why revival meetings produce such an outpouring of changed hearts. All the great speakers pump you up and make you feel like you really can move forward with your wants and desires. In attaching an emotion to an idea for the purpose of motivation, the stronger the emotion, the more compelling the idea (whether it makes sense to anyone else or not).

A fanatic is a prime example of someone who has taken this very concept to an extreme. Tying strong emotions to compelling ideas will produce a relentless person. All the powerful leaders of history felt very ,very strongly about an idea. What makes them so strong is that they were able, through a wide variety of methods, the most common of which being oratory, to transfer their emotional feelings about an idea to their followers. The stronger the feelings, the more fervent the followers, until at last you have the true believer.

But what does all this have to do with THE FABULOUS SEX ORGAN DIET? Just this; you can give yourself a much greater chance of lasting success if, while you are in the process of dropping weight, you become very emotional about your need to do it, to keep doing it, and to finally get it done no matter what. There are two methods of doing this, and you should use both. The first is to get so worked up, whether it's in disgust or some other powerful emotion, that you get to the point where you're absolutely so fed up (no pun intended), that you can't stand it a minute longer. This gets your motivation level so high that the follow through is tremendous.

The second method is more subtle but every bit as

powerful over time. It is the method used by the astronauts, Superbowl and Olympic athletes, and professional musicians, among others, and involves visualizing processes and outcomes. The very best method for producing lasting change is a combination of both A and B. While the first method gives you the power of the charge, the second gives you the ability to refine and adapt!

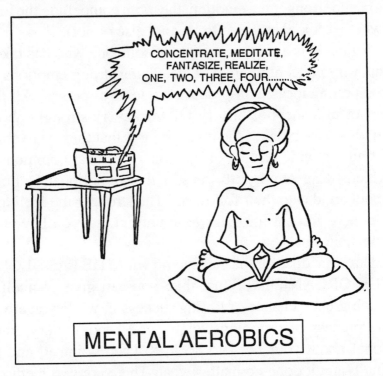

The aforementioned professionals have long used visualization to practice whatever they need to either learn or get better at. Why? Because it has been established by overwhelming evidence that WE BECOME THAT WHICH WE THINK ABOUT! Top professionals have learned to practice their moves or whatever else it is they're trying to accomplish, in their minds when they cannot, for whatever reason, do it in actuality.

So how do we use this to our advantage? Very simply. Whenever you have free moments during the day, or when you're doing something that is easily handled by your autopilot (like driving long distances), visualize in the clearest and most graphic detail of which you are capable, every aspect of your day (or night) that relates to reducing your inventory (losing weight), and see it happening the way you ideally would like it to happen. Pay particular attention to the start and the finish of the said event or events.

As an example, if you're in the habit of going the fridge late at night and grabbing something to eat, you don't have to necessarily erase the entire event, although you certainly can if you wish. But it might be easier in the beginning to twist a habit to do your bidding, rather than try to eliminate it altogether. Picture yourself going to the fridge just like you always do. But instead of grabbing a bunch of food, see yourself looking in there and not really wanting anything to eat tonight. Feel it as you think it! Then, see yourself closing the fridge and walking away perfectly contented, not really in the mood to eat and satisfied that you didn't.

You certainly aren't limited to visualizations about eating. Think about such things as getting ready to exercise. Instead of seeing yourself blowing it off, see yourself deciding to do it. Think about how good you're going to feel when you've finished. Visualize it and feel it!

Another key benefit to visualization is that you can edit current activities to reflect the way you'd prefer they went, instead of the way they've been going. We run pictures and videos through our minds constantly. It's one of the ways we think. What I do when a visualization creeps onto my mental screen that I want to change, rather than trying not to think about it (which as you know is next to impossible, try not to think of a big gray elephant!), I first put a frame around the picture I don't want, then I draw a great big bold X right through the middle of picture to each corner of the frame, and finally have this neat little ol' guy, maybe in a painter's outfit, with a great big bushy mustache, push on the right side of the frame, like it's sitting on a stage, and push it right across the stage and off the screen. Then I immediately visualize the video short the way I really want it to go. Believe me, this stuff really works. The way you are right now is a product of all the ways you see yourself. Change the way you see yourself and you'll win the war!

THE ANAL POWER TECHNIQUE

There are many times during the day when we have free moments for our visualizations. The problem is that there are so many things pulling on our minds, demanding our thoughts, that it's hard to remember to take the time to actually do that which will save us. Believe me, I've been at this for a very long time and I can tell you that if you don't have a regular time set aside every day, you probably won't form the habit of projecting the future of your diet, unless you become so emotionally charged that you think of little else. But even if you have reached the perpetually charged state, the next technique will be very helpful for refining and perfecting your mission.

As I just mentioned, the problem with trying to find a regular time every day, especially if you're a business person or have kids (and if you're a business person with kids you can almost forget it), is that unless you are a very regimented person (in which case I'm sure everything is probably already happening just the way you want it), there is almost no time that isn't already spoken for.

There is at least one time every day that we all have available and it just so happens that it's perfect. Interestingly, George S. Kaufman, one of the most successful and prolific playwrights in the history of Broadway, was also an avid bridge player who did not suffer incompetent players gladly. One day he had a particularly inept player as a partner. This fellow, as the story goes, asked to be excused in order to go to the men's room, to which Kaufman replied, "Gladly -- for the first time today I'll know what you have in your hand."

The point of this little anecdote is to illustrate the extent to which all humans are on automatic pilot when taking a dump. Unless you've got big bowel problems, your experience is very similar to virtually everyone else's in the civilized world. Usually we go at least once a day and, while we're going, there is very little else to do until the job is done (and remember, the job isn't done until the paperwork is out of the way).

What you want to do is find a comfortable position, close your eyes and quickly relax your entire body. The way to do this is to imagine a circle of white light starting at your head and proceeding down your body to your feet. Imagine and feel each part of your body relaxing as the circle of light passes it.

Now that you're relaxed, quickly think of three or four different events that you know will happen or that you want to happen. The important thing is to visualize your specific actions within the episode and imagine them exactly as you would like them to be. This is your time to key your inventory control computer and set the program governing your activities. It's also important to note that no law requires you to instantly spring up and finish the paperwork once you've finished the process of elimination. If you're not finished with your visualizations, finish them first. This way, not only will the movement you're having be smooth, but if used properly, this event could make you a force to be reckoned with.

There are some other reasons, from an anal standpoint, why this time works well. The most important of which is that there are a jumble of emotions swirling around the bowel movement. These emotions often stem from toilet training and the angst one feels at the possibility of no movement when movement is demanded. The bulk of these cross currents from your early childhood were precipitated by your Senior Loan Officer and Waiter.

This S.L.O.W. person was at the heart of most of what went on in your early life, and as they struggled to keep up with your many demands, they had a few of their own, some of which could be responsible for your current troubles. One of them might have been, "Sit there until you go!" The angst comes because you cannot go, yet you must go. The fear is of course, if you don't go, your frustrated banker/caregiver might just cut you off at the knees and leave you feeling like a failure. The interesting thing is that even though you've forgiven and forgotten long ago, those feelings of angst have probably never been erased!

These stored emotions not only haven't left you (it doesn't matter if you no longer actually feel these things about your banker every time you take a dump, according to Freud and many others like him, they're there), and may

UNDERSTANDING THE TECHNOLOGY

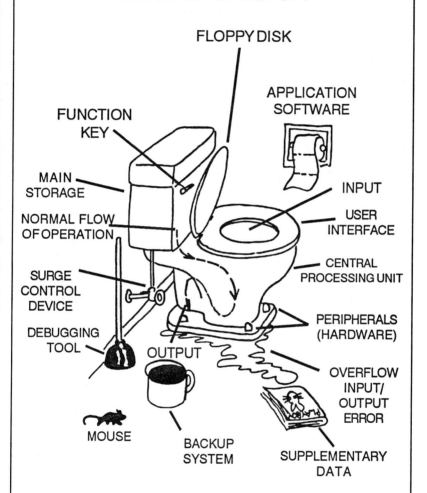

FLOPPY DISK

APPLICATION SOFTWARE

FUNCTION KEY

MAIN STORAGE

INPUT

USER INTERFACE

NORMAL FLOW OF OPERATION

CENTRAL PROCESSING UNIT

SURGE CONTROL DEVICE

DEBUGGING TOOL

OUTPUT

PERIPHERALS (HARDWARE)

OVERFLOW INPUT/ OUTPUT ERROR

MOUSE

BACKUP SYSTEM

SUPPLEMENTARY DATA

ANAL POWER TECHNIQUE -
AS MODERN AS THE COMPUTER AGE

finally have a useful purpose. We can harness the strength of these repressed emotions to enhance the strength of our visualizations! As we succeed in tying an emotion to an idea, our goal becomes a powerful mission that must be accomplished. The ANAL POWER TECHNIQUE can bring your goal to fruition! While it's not well understood in western culture (except of course in San Francisco), THE ANAL POWER TECHNIQUE is rapidly changing the way we think about the way we stink!

CONCLUSION

In conclusion, the body, and THE LIFEFORCE which motivates it, is one of the most profound miracles in all of nature. The mind, of which we use only a fraction, is capable of controlling so many processes that we must conclude it has the ability to control our weight. What we need to do to get it to do our bidding is to set our TIC (thermostat/inventory control) before attempting our big change. The most powerful way to effect a permanent change is to tie a strong emotion to an appealing idea, and then reinforce it with constant visualizations. The very best time to do our visualizations is when we're taking a dump. The reasons are clear. Being regular helps to insure that you aren't overtaken by slip ups late at night. But more importantly, it's a chance to harness any repressed angst that may still may be lingering from a bygone era and use it to emotionally charge an appealing idea.

THE ANAL POWER TECHNIQUE IS A REVOLUTIONARY WAY TO EFFECT THE CHANGES NECESSARY TO BRING YOUR LIFE INTO CONGRUENCE WITH YOUR WANTS AND DESIRES. IT HAS THE ADDED BENEFIT OF ENABLING YOU TO DISCHARGE THAT WHICH YOU MAY BE HARBORING AGAINST THE S.L.O.W. PERSON WHO'S JOB IT WAS TO SEE TO IT THAT YOU BECAME REGULAR WITH YOUR CONTRIBUTION.

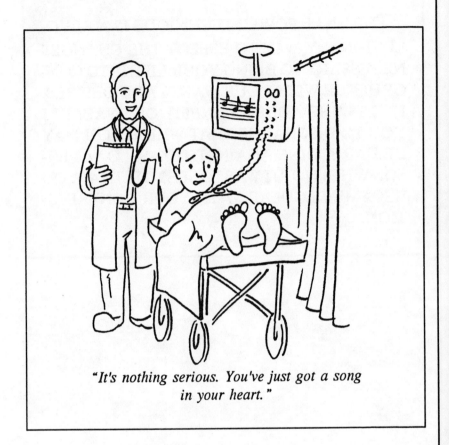

"It's nothing serious. You've just got a song
in your heart."

Chapter 2 -
WHY FAILURES SUCCEED...

It would be easy to begin this chapter on goal setting by reciting reams of platitudes stressing the importance of clearly defining exactly what you want to do before setting out to do it, but I believe that to do so would be a waste of your time. In living my life I've discovered, as you probably have as well, that there is a big gap between advice and help. For that reason I've decided to forego raining down advice from my ivory tower, which isn't necessarily as pristine I would like. Instead, what I'm going to do is help you carry your bundle down the trail, rather than give you a sermon on hiking.

The first thing we need to do is to kick around the most dreaded concept in mainstream Americana; FAILURE. Now there's a chance that if you're reading this book, you have failed in your stated objective to lose weight at least once in your life. Lucky is the soul who happened upon this book before ever attempting a diet, because this will be one of those things in life you won't have to fail at.

But for the rest of you diet hikers that failed for one of a bevy of reasons such as: you got a stone in your shoe and had to stop, you got tired and stopped for a rest, or maybe an unforeseen circumstance got you off the trail. You might be a great starter but a poor finisher. Or maybe, you've tried and failed so much, that you just can't help but think in terms of failure, even though your desire is so strong you can't stop dieting. Do you often, and sometimes even unconsciously, find yourself visualizing the outcome as another failed attempt on your part, even while you're working hard to actually make it happen! If that's the case, you've unknowingly been setting your TIC. Due to the fact that your mind has the power to bring about that which you constantly think about and visualize, your input into your auto-pilot has taken you to failure like a magnet to steel.

If any of the above reasons strike you as a plausible explanation for why you've gotten off the trail, you can finally relax. The aforementioned reasons for failure are so common to the human condition that you should probably give yourself a break, starting immediately! From this point forward, you should cease to think of yourself as some kind of putrid scum, fouling up the earth and choking off humanity in a sea of wretched slime, because you happened to fail in your earlier attempts at weight loss.

Failure is much closer to the essence of the universe than success will ever be. Murphy's Law, which states "what can go wrong, will go wrong," has been proven time and again, by many of our greatest successes, including the late Thomas Alva Edison, who turned failure into an artform. If anything, Edison would probably contend that Murphy was an optimist, and yet Edison was probably the most successful inventor (with the possible exception of Ben Franklin) in the history of our great country!

Why is a man such as Edison, who failed even more times than even Abraham Lincoln (Some of Lincoln's failures are listed below) considered such a great success? It is because he realized that failure is so integral to the process of success, that you literally cannot have success without it.

Lincoln's Adult Life
1831 - Failed in business
1832 - Defeated in a bid for the Illinois legislature
1833 - Death of Ann Rutledge
1834 - Second failure in business
1836 - Suffered a nervous breakdown
1838 - Defeated in bid for speaker of the Illinois house
1840 - Defeated in bid for being a Whig elector
1848 - Defeated in bid for the U.S. House of Representatives
1855 - Defeated in a bid for U.S. Senate
1856 - Defeated in a bid for the Republican vice-presidential nomination
1858 - Again defeated in a bid for the U.S. Senate
1860 - Elected President of the United States

Failure is one side of a coin we call trial and error, and it's usually the result of either doing something the wrong way, or not doing it long enough the right way, to finally make it work. All the truly successful human beings in history (and please note this includes men) have met with many more failures than the average dieter.

The reason these failures didn't stop, and as a consequence went on to succeed, is that it never occurred to them that failure was a permanent condition.

Consider this, just as it is critically important in the rearing of children to distinguish between the child and his actions; i.e. telling children that they are bad, is simply not as productive as telling them that even though what they did was bad, they remain good kids. It is essential to make the same distinction for yourself. By doing this, both you and the kids will continue to see yourselves as basically good, which keeps your auto-pilot steering both of you in the right direction.

We, as presumably older and wiser individuals, must make the same distinction in our attempt to accomplish our goals here on the planet. Just as there is a huge difference between being broke and being poor, there is a great expanse between failing at things we've attempted, and being failures as human beings!

Remember; the only time you can't afford to fail is the last time you try!

Another reason, and probably the more important of the two, is that successful people succeed because they are on a mission so vitally important (at least in their mind) that they will let nothing stand in the way of its accomplishment. It almost sounds like they're relentless, doesn't it?

In short, successful people are people who successfully link a strong feeling or emotion to an idea they have to accomplish. This gives them the power to transcend failure and become relentless in their drive to success! We discussed this technique in the last chapter in conjunction with making important changes in our lives. But it is essential that we employ this powerful technique not only to change our lives by creating DEFINING MO-

CHAPTER 2

MENTS, but to eradicate the destructive feelings that are brought on by the inability to put failure into perspective. To become relentless, we must use all the tools in our toolbox!

Even if you've failed as a dieter more than a thousand times and feel as though there is no hope for ever becoming skinny, let me remind you that Edison tried ten thousand different materials before he came up with the idea of using cotton thread for the filament in his first lightbulb. Ten thousand! And while we obviously can't all be Edisons, we can become Edisonsque. Which simply means, that we can emulate the qualities of Edison that we feel will be valuable in producing success in our own lives.

The most important of which, as I just mentioned, is becoming relentless in the pursuit of what you want. Once you become relentless, failures (yes, you'll still have them) will become minor setbacks. They'll become no more than bumps in the road. You'll notice them and be disappointed by them as is only natural. But you're certainly not going to stop the car because of them. When you adopt this mindset, failure becomes irrelevant, because you're going to do what it takes, regardless! As you surely know, when you're bound and determined to do something, dammit you're going to do it, and that's all there is to it!

I'll give you a classic example of just exactly what I mean. A very good friend of mine, Terry , came very close to cashing in his chips with a sudden heart problem and had to have major bypass surgery, like right now. Did it scare him? You bet! So when the doctor told him he was fifty pounds over weight and had to lose it, do you think he said, "Gee Doc I don't know, I've tried losing weight but it just won't come off." Heck no! The strength of the emotions he experienced when confronted with death were very strong, as you might expect, and were easily tied to the idea of slimming down. Needless to say, he became relentless. He lost the weight and is now healthier than he's ever been, with the possible exception of his heart, of course.

In short, Terry became a man on a mission, and failure never even entered his mind. It wasn't even a consideration. He was bound and determined to finally do what he had been trying to do for years but could never quite manage, and he did it. Fortunately, we don't need to stare death in the face to become bound and determined. When you've finished with this book you'll realize that it's within your power to become relentless, and if you decide to do so, you will be successful. The point of the illustration, however, is simply to demonstrate that no matter how many times you've failed to lose weight in the past, either because you got started and then quit or because you talked about it but never even got started, it just doesn't matter! If you take the time to use the ANAL POWER TECHNIQUE, eat your sex organs every day, and hook up the Pre D-Day Attitude Adaptor explained in chapter 6, you will be relentless. And when you become relentless, YOU SUCCEED!

BENEFITS

Now that we've pretty much eliminated the possibility of failure, and before we get to the heart of the FABULOUS SEX ORGAN DIET, let's explore some of the more obvious benefits of succeeding in reducing your inventories by adjusting your TIC, so that your Corporation of Cells will start using "just in time inventories" and keep you skinny.

I hope that by now you're starting to get personally excited about your prospects. If you're not, you should be, because opportunity is knocking. Eating raw sex organs every day isn't a right, it's a privilege! You can have that privilege if it's important to you to "regroove" and get on a better track than the one you're on.

I ate my sex organs today and I feel great. That feeling is one of the supreme benefits of eating sex organs. You get tremendous energy. Do you want to be a human dynamo? Well here's your chance. Sex organs contain not only life giving energy, but the very essence of life itself, and your body hungers for it.

Imagine, for a moment, waking up early every morning refreshed, with the feeling that you're ready to take on the world. You're clear headed, with no grogginess and you feel no inclination to languish in bed to get those last few precious minutes of sleep. You're up, you're alive, and you're beaming around the house thinking of all the things you can't wait to do. Why? Because you've been filling yourself with THE LIFEFORCE found in sex organs and, you're so excited, you're telling everyone - and they're listening!

Now after reading that, but having yet to experience it, you're probably thinking, "He's full of something alright..." and you're probably right, but that's beside the point. Once you start gorging yourself on sex organs every morning, the life in your body will energize before your very eyes and quite frankly, I think you'll be shocked at how much there is left. The important thing to do at this point is to sit back and spend a moment fertilizing your fantasy with visualization. Why not? What do you have to lose? What do you want to lose? If your body has been yearning for more than you're getting, the time has come to go get it!

The next benefit is, in the minds of many, even more exciting than having the dynamic feeling of abundant energy without having to drink tons of coffee. This benefit is of course tremendous sex appeal. If you don't want sex appeal, you should be prepared to wear layer upon layer of heavy clothing, including the possible use of mosquito netting, to obscure the evidence that THE LIFEFORCE is exuding from you.

I've known women who didn't want to have sex appeal. In fact, they gained weight just so they didn't have to deal with the inevitable lust their body was likely to inspire. Feeling uncomfortable with the lust that sex appeal inspires, is a tough one. I myself find it difficult to deal with, but we've all got to make sacrifices. When you're fat, everyone likes you for your wonderful personality, right? But lose the weight, and now on top of that wonderful personality that you've taken so much pride in all these years, you've got something that is almost certain to inspire carnal thoughts in the minds of others.

Question; Do you go from being a warm, wonderful person, to a warm, wonderful person with increased sex appeal after you SLIM DOWN, TONE UP and begin exuding THE LIFEFORCE? Could you stand it if you did?

Katherine Whitehorn once observed that outside every thin woman is a fat man trying to get in, and she's probably right. Sex is the most dominant force on earth. It has inspired all of the oldest professions and has fostered many a growth industry. It is the single biggest factor in advertising. In fact, there is very little that isn't advertised using a blatant attempt to get one's product linked subliminally to a lusty hard body.

Does that make sex dirty? Only if it's done right. The lust we feel is a chemically induced reaction to a healthy visual stimulus. Unfortunately, there is no way to determine (even by using modern scientists of both sexes, half clothed, and studying furiously), whether lust is good for you or whether it simply leads to profound hair growth on the palms. I truly believe that the biggest problem with having tremendous sex appeal, is being thought of as little more than a sex object while many of your other fine qualities go completely unnoticed. If this is your problem believe me, I understand, because it happens to me all the time and I hate feeling like just another piece of hot molten flesh.

But if you decide that you love all the energy you're getting from your daily ingestion of sex organs, the fact is you're going to have to live with all the lust you're likely to inspire as a result of not only your wonderful vivaciousness, but because of your new found shapeliness.

Now granted this new found shapeliness is going to take a little time, but the reason time was created in the first place was so that everything didn't happen all at once. Can you imagine how miserable life would be if every thing didn't take time? There'd be no need to string people along or procrastinate for even a minute, and then where would we be? We'd be forced to deal with everything RIGHT NOW, and sometimes things just take a little time. So let's be eternally thankful that this is going to take some time (but it won't be as much as you think!). While you're not going to be a skinny drink of water overnight, it's best to start thinking about it right away.

Question; Why is it that we never have the time to do it right, but we always have time to do it over?

There is another benefit that you may or may not want, so you should be aware of it, in order to take effective counter measures if necessary. While it remains undocumented in the strict scientific sense (which is the sense that you can never get scientists to agree on virtually anything, except of course on how to build a Hubble telescope) there is anecdotal evidence that a healthy diet of sex organs can significantly increase your virility or fertility, depending on the nature of your plumbing and your outlook on life.

Take me for example, I have been unable, up until recently, when I had my works cut out for me, to stop making embryos. I remember the first time I got my wife pregnant. She went to the doctor and he said," Mama, it looks like twins." So she came home and told me and I said," That's wonderful, what do you think we ought to name them?" She said," Adolf and Rudolph." Ten months later she's pregnant again. She went to the doctor and again it looked like twins. She came home and told me, and naturally I was ecstatic. I asked her what we should name them. She said, "Getoff and Stayoff."

So there you have it, our dilemma. My wife was pregnant a total of three times in twenty-seven months (we had been married only slightly longer than that). The pill failed us. We tried using the diaphragm, but because it's a new and complex technology, I could never figure out which went in

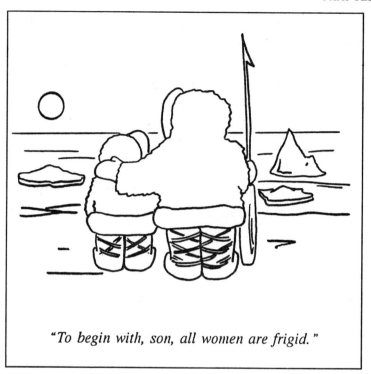

"To begin with, son, all women are frigid."

first, me or the diaphragm. The third time, two weeks after my wife has an IUD installed at the garage, she became pregnant again! Let me tell you what, having this many kids this quickly is like having a bowling alley installed in your brain, with leagues running night and day. So do be careful with THE LIFEFORCE!!

Before I talk further about the possibility of improving your fertility, I should mention that since being put on temporary overload as a direct result of my good fortune to have so many wonderful little babies all at once, I've been telling friends who are considering the stygian crossing, that they shouldn't begin having kids until right near the end of their life. That way, once you realize that life as you know it is over, it won't matter as much.

When I was a kid, my dad gave me a piece of advice that I should have taken to heart. He said, "John, do you know the reason I only had two kids? It was because I read somewhere that every third person born was a chinaman, and at the time I didn't want no Chinese for a kid." Well exceeding dad's limit on children didn't produce an oriental child, but it did make me wonder if I shouldn't take it easy on the sex organs every morning.

Here's another example of why kids can be so much fun. A while back, my small son gets up and comes downstairs to get ready for day school. I asked him, "Brett, what would you like for breakfast?" He says, much to my surprise, "Give me some of those damned corn flakes." In my shock, I knocked him upside the head and asked him again, "What do you want for breakfast?" Again he spurts out, "I want some of those damned corn flakes!" This time I really let him have it, and when I finally asked him for a third time what he wanted for breakfast, he says to me, "Well, you can bet your ass it won't be corn flakes!" Kids...

With that in mind, let me briefly sum up the argument for having no more than two kids with a great poem from ages past...

> There once was a girl who begat
> Three babies named Nat, Pat, and Tat
> It was fun in the breeding
> But hell in the feeding
> When she found there was no tit for Tat!

Seriously, I believe the case to be made for increased fertility lies in the body's ability to work toward perfect health when given the chance. As we have already seen, the mind has the ability to control a level of complexity that man himself can not begin to comprehend. This control mechanism constantly compares and contrasts the body's current state of health with the ideal and attempts to bring them into line. If it's true (and the evidence seems to indicate that it is) that eating life giving, life sustaining, and life restoring sex organs aids the body in its quest for perfect health, then shouldn't you eat them as a matter of course? You will find that eating sex organs every morning, as per THE FABULOUS SEX ORGAN DIET, will make you feel healthier! If you desire to improve the possibility of increasing your fertility, you should of course consult with your physician or faith healer.

For me to assert that there is a direct relationship between THE FABULOUS SEX ORGAN DIET and increased fertility is, naturally outrageous. All I can say is, PLEASE don't underestimate the effect THE LIFEFORCE can have on your life!

In chapter 5 we will further explore how many of the things we ingest are often laced with things we generally don't want to know about. There is no telling how much of what we eat affects our organs. Unlike engine parts that can be removed and examined for the harmful buildup of deposits, we haven't yet gotten to that point with our own organs. So remember, until further notice, the only place you should leave deposits is in a financial institution, because when they build up in the body, trouble begins.

CONCLUSION

Please remember that it makes absolutely no sense to beat up on yourself for failures and mistakes of the past. Knocking yourself in the side of the head all the time because you aren't pleased with your conduct will only make you dizzy. Give yourself a break, and remember that the greatest people in history failed at things they attempted all the time. They simply were far too relentless to let a temporary setback stop them from doing what they decided to do.

To succeed, we too must become relentless!

Finally, filling your body with THE LIFEFORCE (and we're about to find out how), will have long range cosmic effects on your health and your mental feeling of well being. Whether eating sex organs every morning will lead to an increase in your fertility or not, is open to debate. But what isn't open for debate is that your body can do remarkable things, and it's short sighted to be less than optimistic about what you are truly capable of when you put your mind to it!

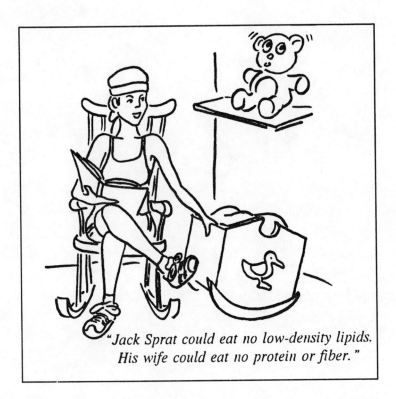

"*Jack Sprat could eat no low-density lipids.
His wife could eat no protein or fiber.*"

Chapter 3 -
THE HEART OF THE DIET,
SEX ORGANS IN A NUT SHELL (for protection)

The body uses a certain amount of energy every day to conduct its business. This energy can be gotten from either ingested food or stored reserves (fat). The secret to gaining weight, which is probably no secret at all, is to take in more energy in the form of food than you can burn up. If you do this, those little storage facilities we call fat cells will fill up in no time. Once all the pre-existing fat cells in the body are full, your body will build new ones to hold all the inventory you seem to keep ordering.

To lose weight, all you need to do is burn up more energy every day than you're taking in. This way, inventories will be used to supply your factory with fuel. As these inventories are reduced, all those little collapsible warehouses the body built for storage will shrink and finally waste away, once it's obvious to the body that they won't be refilled again. As this happens, you get lighter.

Sounds easy doesn't it? All you do is dramatically reduce your intake and viola! You're suddenly lighter. But it isn't that simple for a simple reason. We have a very complex security system to protect us from ourselves. It acts not only to maintain the TIC setting (Temperature/Inventory Control), but has a little paranoia meter that sends off an alarm when one's self preservation is somehow threatened. When the alarm goes off, the security force will react with countermeasures, and the magnitude of these measures will depend on the extent of the perceived threat.

That's why "low calorie" diets are doomed to failure unless you become a complete masochist. These diets seem to work at first, but it's only because your security force will make an extra effort to use food still laying in the intestines, giving you the appearance of weight loss. But they ultimately fail because once the blood sugar level falls below a certain point, countermeasures will definitely kick in.

You may find this hard to believe, but the body has a morbid fear of starving to death. When the body starts feeling like it might be starving, it has the security force instruct each cell in the body to immediately begin burning less. So the net effect is, that while you're doing all this suffering, trying to starve yourself thin, the security force is busy trying to cut you off at the pass, cell by cell. This is a very difficult fight to win!

Along with the ability to dramatically reduce your overall metabolism in an attempt to thwart the starvation threat, your body can produce the feeling of an insane hunger for that which can be converted into blood sugar very quickly. Take a guess what that is!?! You got it: cakes, pies, cookies, rolls, donuts, chips, pop, ice cream, candy bars, and a wide variety of fast foods.

Since hunger is almost certainly one of the most reliable of sensations the body can produce, let's see how it's triggered. Each of us has in our brain, a blood sugar or glucose detector located in the hypothalamus. One of several important reasons why the brain is concerned about the blood sugar level in the body is that glucose is all the brain can use for energy. The brain will actually short the rest of the body in emergencies so that it can keep functioning. For this reason, a body running low on blood sugar is like a donut shop running out of flour! Something's got to be done right now.

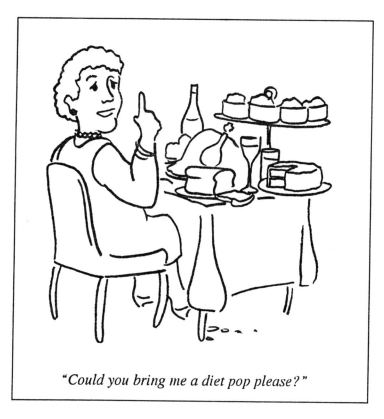

"Could you bring me a diet pop please?"

So when our blood sugar falls below a certain point, we get an unpleasant feeling that we've learned to associate with the need to eat. The hunger trigger works something like the gadget that controls the water level in your toilet. When the sugar level drops below a certain point, the alarm goes off and sends you a memo, like phone mail. As the level continues to drop, the messages get more urgent, like closed door sessions with the boss. When you get totally starved, as in, "I could eat a horse," the corporate culture begins to turn on you and you don't have a friend anywhere in the body until you get your blood sugar up.

Interestingly enough, the shut off switch seems to be based on a net percentage increase in the blood sugar (the amount it increases from the low point) rather than total blood sugar. That's why when you eat out and order half the menu because you feel so starved (hoping some of it comes right away, and the rest follows soon after), you're shocked when you can't eat even half of what you ordered. We use expressions like, "My eyes were bigger than my stomach" or "My stomach must have shrunk" to explain this experience. But the truth is you raised your blood sugar enough with your initial intake to turn off the switch.

So, in essence, trying to starve yourself skinny pits your conscious mind against a very elaborate security system that controls your primal feelings, like hunger and thirst. This system can literally take control of your actions and motivate you to act in ways IT perceives as being in your best interest. When you pit the forces of nature within you against your conscious mind, unless you are Herculean, your conscious mind has very little chance!

When you don't understand what you're actually up against, you can't possibly understand why you failed! Repeatedly failing often leads low self esteem and self worth, and generally promotes bad psychology, especially if you attempt to mentally minimize the strength of the forces aligned against your effort. Let me make it very clear to you once and for all -- the primal forces that control your base drives and survival instincts are some of the strongest forces known to exist on earth. Therefore, if you want to be effective in your effort to lose weight, you must first get in harmony with your system, do not battle with it! To lose weight, you don't use will power, but you must use your mind power. Only through the power that you've been given to reset and reprogram your TIC can you get your system to do your bidding, instead of giving you another beating.

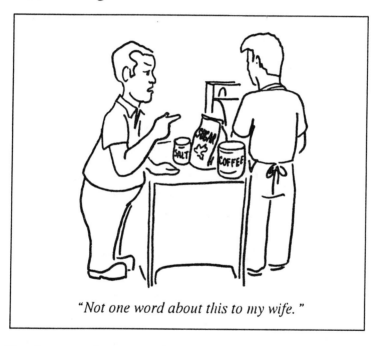

"Not one word about this to my wife."

By the way, just as a side bar, this is the same principle for quitting any habit you may have acquired that your security force has an interest in preserving. Willpower usually isn't enough, because you don't have enough of the troops on your side. Marshall your forces first, by resetting your TIC with the Anal Power Technique, and you'll find that all of a sudden, as Jimmy Stewart would say, "It's A

Wonderful Life"

In order to help you see the total beauty and simplicity of THE FABULOUS SEX ORGAN DIET, I've been trying to lay enough ground work for you to understand how utterly congruous it is with your body. For that reason I want to delve into the operation of the body's refueling system before going any further. The more you understand about how it works, the more you'll be impressed by just how cosmic THE FABULOUS SEX ORGAN DIET really is. The more impressed you are, the easier it will be for you to use it to your advantage.

Eating...

First, let's understand that your body will only produce so much energy on any given day. It's how you use this energy that determines what you actually get done during your waking hours. The single biggest use the body has for this energy is operating the digestive system. It uses more energy than running, swimming, or even biking. The process involves a rather large list of component operations. It starts with the arms shoveling the food in (I'm not even mentioning preparation)... The jaw chewing, while the salivary glands under the tongue pump out saliva (and your glands use a lot of energy), and then more muscles take the food, chew by chew, down to that cavernous pit you call a stomach.

In the stomach are a number of glands. Some that secrete acid and some that produce enzymes to further break down what has just been chewed. Depending upon how heavy the food and extensive the intake, the glands in your stomach may have to duke it out with the load you shoveled in for as long as eight hours. The stomach's extensive use of the glucose in the blood stream to get this job done can, and often does, leave the rest of the body short. The brain will create a feeling of tiredness to slow the body down (in order to preserve available blood sugar), until more can be obtained from the digestive process itself.

Once the stomach has done all it can do, muscle action pushes this digested material (the name for this material is chyme and is pronounced -- "kime") through a thirty foot tube we call the intestines. In the intestines, further digestion takes place. (As an example, fats are emulsified with bile in the section of intestine immediately following the stomach).

The main event however, is the absorption of all that the body needs to operate. These nutrients are absorbed into the blood stream via numerous small projections, sticking out about a quarter of an inch from the intestinal wall, called villi. Think of the inside of the intestine as being lined with something resembling medium pile carpeting. Your muscles must push the chyme through this carpet for thirty feet. It's just not easy! It takes strong muscles hours and hours to get the job done.

The last four or five feet of the intestine is referred to as the large intestine. It's here that the body gets the scrap ready for shipment. This tube is the big compactor. As it compacts material, it also wrings out the excess water still remaining. Finally, when the time is right, it facilitates the not always quick, and not always easy, process of elimination. All this work takes tremendous energy. One of the things that THE FABULOUS SEX ORGAN DIET does for you is to help reduce substantially the amount of energy required for digestion, absorption, and elimination, leaving more energy for the things you want to do on your own.

Think of the utilization of energy to complete the digestive process this way. Imagine you're on a vacation, and you have budgeted two hundred dollars a day for everything you want to do. You know that you have to eat and sleep somewhere. If you check into the most expensive place in town, where the rooms are $150 a night, and you spend $40 a day to eat, you don't have a hell of a lot left to do all the things you've planned. But if you stay at a place that's every bit as nice but only costs you $70 per night, all of a sudden you have all kinds of money to spend. Your vacation is a lot more fun because you can do a whole lot more.

The same holds true for you and the total amount of energy you have available every day to do all that you and your body have planned! If you only have a certain amount of energy available to you every day (no matter how much you overeat), and a large percentage of that is used just to process the incoming fuel, the amount you have left determines, to a large extent, how you feel. You can't possibly have the boundless energy to do all the things you want to do, if your digestive system has just sucked you dry!

When you lose this energy, guess what happens! You feel sluggish. When you get sluggish, your motivation level drops substantially! As your motivation level plunges, some of what you had in mind to do will almost certainly get sacrificed. As a consequence, you tend to lounge more and more, which means that you'll burn even less. When you don't burn your daily quota of liquid energy, it gets stored as inventory, warehoused as fat somewhere in the body.

So by reducing the amount of energy it takes to digest food, you increase the energy available to the rest of the body. This will have an immediate impact on your motivation level. When you feel full of energy, you're going to be up zipping around, not lounging around! The true beauty of this is that not only do you start to feel like you're getting more done every day and taking charge of your life, but when you are up zipping around, burning more than you're taking in, what happens? That's right, you lose weight!

I want to spend a moment on coffee and caffeine while we're on the subject of energy. Coffee is easily one of the most popular drinks in the world and is in no danger of losing that status. If for no other reason than the fact that it's a great social lubricant, coffee will be with us always-"Let's go get a cup of coffee," is one of America's finest lines. Coffee's most popular attribute is, almost without question, it's ability to get caffeine quickly into the blood stream, giving one a feeling of increased energy. People love stimulants because they produce in us a heightened state, that enables us to be more efficient. But there are some side effects to caffeine intake that tend to subvert the weight loss process.

When you put caffeine into your system, it gives you the feeling of increased energy and heightened awareness by inducing the body to increase its production of adrenalin. After the initial surge you feel upon ingestion, the central nervous system metabolizes the remainder at a steady rate until it's gone. Unlike eating something high in refined sugar, like a donut, where the blood sugar spikes and then trails off, caffeine's effect is continuous. But when it's gone, suddenly it's all gone!

What you don't feel is the adrenalin indirectly stimulating the pancreas to dramatically increase the production of insulin. Insulin is the bridge that enables sugar to get from the blood to the cells of the body that need it. A spike in insulin production has the effect of sharply dropping the blood sugar. Caffeine camouflages this drop while it remains in the body by reducing or eliminating the feeling of hunger.

If you try to lose weight by simultaneously reducing your food intake and increasing your caffeine consumption, you might think you're fooling your body, but in reality, your body is actually fooling you. The reason is that if the blood sugar level gets low enough, the brain will signal the body to begin dissolving your muscles to get available protein, which it will then turn into sugar through a process known as gluconeogenesis. The problem with losing weight by dissolving your muscles is, since muscles burn the bulk of all the energy used in the body, over time, your body will burn less and less of what you eat. As a result, it becomes even more difficult to even stay at the weight you were at before you started.

After the caffeine has been entirely metabolized, you will feel an immediate and sometimes sharp, drop in your energy level. This drop will make you feel tired and worn out, almost immediately. You get a spent feeling (especially if you've been drinking it all day), leaving you just enough strength to make it to the couch or the easy chair for a little rest, at least that's the way it starts. But unfortunately, that's where you die for the next several hours until the body recoups.

Needless to say, your motivation level at this point is so

low that life is temporarily put on hold until you sleep. This down and dirty energy drop that occurs as the caffeine is finally completely metabolized within the body is what I refer to as "Coffee Burn." The disappointing thing about having this is, if it happens in conjunction with filling up on dinner, you'll be forced to labor under the almost impossible weight of both the coffee burn and the tired feeling you probably get from eating dinner. If this is happening to you, you're forcing your body to warehouse a ton of inventory, and it's hard to get thin when you're filling your storage facilities every night!!

There are other problems with caffeine that are a little more insidious but every bit as destructive to your well being. Prolonged use of caffeine has the same effect, albeit to a lesser extent, as the regular use of cocaine, speed, or any of the more serious stimulants that people enjoy taking for various purposes. It causes the depletion of neurotransmitters and ion relays in the nervous system. When these are gone, or even substantially reduced, your moods will sink, and they won't recover. The depletion of these neurotransmitters can make you feel like you are literally going insane!

You won't notice it at first, because it's so darned insidious. But as your attitude goes south (if you have eroded your natural ability to deal with stress, your level of paranoia will start to rise)... and gloom will start to hang over you like a cloud! In point of fact, taking too much caffeine over time will leave you with the feeling that life is horseshit, which, as you know, is bullshit. This will become clear to you as you fill yourself with THE LIFEFORCE!

At a particularly disappointing point in my life, a friend of mine, Byron Hosmer ACSW, a psychotherapist, cornered me about all the coffee I was drinking. He suggested that this very action alone could be responsible for my generally sagging mental state. So I completely stopped for two months.

The first thing that happened was that I started going through withdrawal. Can you believe it? This included a constant headache and a pronounced cranky feeling for a week. But after putting that behind me, my feeling of well being began to climb back to the land of the living. After a couple of months I absolutely couldn't believe how thoroughly improved were both my attitude and my feeling of well being.

Upon relaying this to Byron some months later, he told me that he had a similar problem with caffeine and had to give it up altogether. He then told me that he runs across this problem all the time. People who take the cure are shocked at what an effect something as seemingly innocuous as coffee can have. Believe me when I say, the effect that substantial coffee drinking can have on your mental attitude is more significant than you realize! Give your body time to replenish your neurotransmitters by cutting out caffeine, and you'll be glad you did!

By relating this to you I am not on a kick-the-coffee habit soapbox; but you will find that with this diet you really won't need it (this goes as well for all you folks who drink tons of certain soft drinks because its in there too!). In short, it's safe to say that caffeine does quite a few things that have the effect of minimizing your potential in this or any other life. Since being on a diet makes you results oriented almost by default, if you want to improve your results, lighten up on things containing caffeine. I will say, as a bit of encouragement, that once you start gorging yourself on sex organs every morning, you won't even miss it!

The Digestive Cycle

There is a very distinct digestive cycle that our system follows. We need to not only be aware of it, but go as far as we can to facilitate it so that we can maximize our energy gain and weight loss. Let me explain. We do the bulk of all our eating between eleven in the morning and seven at night. This food is then processed and converted into fuel from the time that dinner ends until four or five in the morning. Finally, the process of elimination begins, and fills our morning hours with an opportunity to, among other things, reset our TIC. By augmenting these seemingly routine functions we can help our bodies to get more digesting done and take less energy to do it!

The importance of these components of the digestive cycle must not be underestimated. When you think in terms of your natural daily rhythms, several things will probably pop out at you. First, you probably have a bowel movement (take a dump) before noon. Secondly, while you generally can skip breakfast without much problem, trying to skip lunch is a bear! Finally, you rarely find that you have any interest in a big meal after the early evening time frame. Except of course if you've been out drinking. Drinking alcohol has a tendency to make you arrhythmic.

The schedule of this cycle will obviously be somewhat different for "true" night people. But for the folks who have their rhythms tied to the sun, this is the story. For this reason, the times for beginning and ending individual segments of the overall digestive cycle described in THE FABULOUS SEX ORGAN DIET are designed to enhance and maximize the efficiency of digestive activities based on the daily sun cycle!

The Diet

The time has come to explore the essence of the diet. So let's get down to it, shall we! For our purposes, I'm going to divide the food we eat into two groups and contrary to popular thought, it's not going to be good food and bad food, but rather light foods and heavy foods. The light foods are EDIBLE SEX ORGANS FROM THE PLANT WORLD and vegetables. The importance of these sex organs lies in the fact that they contain the most comic force in the universe -- LIFE!

An edible, life giving sex organ is the fruit of the plant that bore it. A fruit is defined scientifically as: The fertilized ovary of a seed bearing plant, where the seeds are contained inside some sort of pulpy envelope. Furthermore, the fruit is an outgrowth from the flower of the plant. The flower being the device used for the fertilization of this ovary or seed.

This means that scientists include many more things in the category of fruits, than the average consumer. Such things as beans, squash, cucumbers, nuts, tomatoes, peppers, corn, peas, and a host of other things that we generally think of as vegetables are all fruits. Let me further add that the definition of a vegetable is: Any edible part of a plant. This includes roots and tubers, stalks, flowers, buds, stems, leaves, and the fruit of the plant. Scientifically, a fruit is a vegetable, but as you can easily see, most vegetables are not fruits!

The point of eating fruits in the morning to milk their manifold benefits will be discussed in detail over the next several pages. But the very essence of why they are so incredibly beneficial to us is that nature has imbued fruit with a vey high concentration of THE LIFEFORCE. Think about it, these are the reproductive organs that spawn life. They not only spawn life, but they have to do it under some of the most extreme of circumstances. For that reason nature made THE LIFEFORCE very strong in fruits. Fruits contain everything necessary to foster and accelerate the growth of life at a very critical stage in the plant's overall development; that is, before the plant is technically even a plant.

Without a doubt, the beauty of eating the reproductive organs of plants is that you are ingesting that which gives and creates life. Put that life into your body and you become, over time, absolutely full of it! You will be literally imbued with the most cosmic force in the universe. This force will absolutely energize your life if you'll let it!

I just heard something that I think you'll find very interesting, and highlights how this concept is spreading. Wurlitzer is going to merge with Xerox and together they're going to make reproductive organs. However, there is no indication at this early date that they will be included in the FABULOUS SEX ORGAN DIET. I guess there's quite a bit of testing by the FDA that has to happen first. But I'll let you know.

Beyond that, let me say at this point that I hope you're not too terribly disappointed that we aren't talking about consuming the sex organs of various members of the animal kingdom, particularly those of your fellow man. IT IS interesting to note however, that while it isn't the thrust of this book to discuss eatable animal organs, it is worth noting that the way you say vagina in Chinese is "tongue chow" (this is spelled phonetically of course).

So Asia's apparently already on board with the plan. Further, even though research reports are very limited on the matter in China, I think we can safely assume that any group of people who can make several billion kids in their spare time may not need reports. I've been given to understand that the oral tradition is very strong in Asia. By the way, do you like to eat Chinese? If so, you're in luck because that sort of thing is on the diet. Get those salivary glands ready!

Augmenting the natural digestive cycles of the body is done with a water wash every morning using sex organs. The water wash is very important. As I mentioned earlier, the intestines process the digested food coming from the stomach. This stuff looks like a pasty, gooey mass, and flows through the carpet like lining of villi, until it gets absorbed into the system. The problem is, as you can well imagine, some of this goo stays behind, and over time can build up deposits. As an example, it is generally estimated that by the time the average meat eater reaches fifty, they have as much as five pounds of undigested red meat in their intestines. Which, as you might guess, can cause considerable intestinal difficulty over time, as it compacts and decays between the villi. Remember, this has been going on inside you for decades already! Decades!

It's as simple as this: Can you imagine how dirty your kitchen floor would get over time if it were never cleaned? It would be so covered with gunk after a few decades that you probably wouldn't be able to see the linoleum! Fortunately, the body has a process for cleaning up the mess inside you. When you lend a hand (but not a finger) the process becomes even more efficient.

That's why THE FABULOUS SEX ORGAN DIET is so cosmic, on so many different levels! Eating only sex organs every morning (because they're everything you need, without the things you don't need) does a number of very good things at the same time. Fruits are up to 90% water. In fact a ripe tomato can be up to 97% water! The rest is soluble fiber, fructose, a sugar (you might expect that the name of the sugar in a sex organ is frucktose), and multiple vitamins. For these reasons, fruit in the morning is absolutely perfect from an energy, health, and dietary stand point.

When you chew fruit, it is predigested in the mouth by your saliva. As a consequence, it only spends about twenty minutes in the stomach and then proceeds to the intestines. There, the water content washes the tube, while the villi pick up the energy contained in the fructose, and wisp it into the blood supply. This washing does two very important things. First it moves yesterday's waste out the door, so it doesn't hang around and decompose while it's still in you. Second, it washes the villi so that they can do their job more efficiently. It's amazing how much more efficient they are, when they're clean.

What does this efficiency do for you? Ever tried to wipe mud or snow off your feet onto a mat that's already caked with it? Not much gets cleaned off, it just gets moved around. The same thing's true with your intestines. When your body gets all the nutrients it needs to function sooner and quite a bit easier, the hunger alarm gets shut off much earlier into the meal. So you end up eating less to get the same net effect, from both an energy and a "full feeling" standpoint, as you were getting previously.

There are two basic reasons, aside from the need to satisfy one's oral frustrations (which may be molified by cramming sex organs in your mouth), that the body requires one to overeat. The first is due to clogged villi. When the villi get clogged or matted down, the body must cause more material to pass over them so they can absorb all the nutrients needed by the body for its daily operation. The second reason the body will induce you to eat more than you need is that it knows exactly what it does need, in terms of nutrients, to conduct business every day. If it can't get what it needs, it will tell you to keep eating in hopes of finally scoring.

This is why pregnant women often have cravings. When the body has determined that it's not getting enough of a certain nutrient, it will create a hunger for something you've recently eaten that has that nutrient in it, and it'll keep up the desire for that particular food until it gets enough of the particular nutrient. Meanwhile, you may have just eaten a tremendous amount of food to get it! YOU CAN ELIMINATE BOTH THESE PROBLEMS BY EATING ABSOLUTELY NOTHING BUT SEX OR-GANS (FRUIT) BEFORE LUNCH!

The biggest benefit of all has only been touched upon, and that's all the extra energy you have. Look at it this way, if your body doesn't have to waste a great deal of the energy it created from yesterday's intake to digest breakfast alone, you're going to have a great deal of energy left, which at one time you wasted! So you're going to be a highly motivated individual instead of a slug. Furthermore, because of the tremendous volume of liquid energy you're getting from the fruit, you're pumped and primed, and you didn't have to drink a quart of coffee to do it. Coupled with this is the fact that you can't possibly feel hungry eating a bevy of sex organs every morning. The fructose keeps the blood sugar alarm from going off and signaling you to eat more. You won't have the urge to munch down a bevy of donuts (which you're drawn to because your brain needs the sugar) in the morning!

In point of fact, the brain uses two thirds of all the blood sugar in the body. That's why it gets so concerned when the supply gets short. The brain will literally force you to eat things that raise it quickly to insure it's proper functioning. That's why many people feel that sex organs are Brain Food!

At this point I should add that not only are sex organs the ticket to a wonderful feeling of well being, but the juice of sex organs is also great! It's a fabulous sugar filled wash, that kick starts your motor, I mean right now! In fact, that's why the juicier the fruit the better the fruit! Personally, I prefer a couple of lush, firm melons sitting in front of me at the breakfast table, and my wife, bless her heart, sees to it. It's so nice to take them in your hands and feel how wonderful they are as you gorge yourself on their delectability. You're certainly in very little danger of overstuffing yourself with melons, because once you're full of it, and you'll sense when you're full of it, it's pretty much time to shut the ol' trap, don't you think?

We still haven't even talked about the benefit for which all America seems to be craving, and that's soluble fiber! Oats, which as you might have guessed, are not only the source of oatbran (ever hear of that?), but the oat seed is a sex organ that has gained popularity for its ability to reduce fat and cholesterol uptake in the intestines . Do you know what property of the oat seed actually does this for you? It's the soluble fiber! FRUIT HAS TONS OF SOLUBLE FIBER! Soluble fiber substantially limits the uptake of fat and cholesterol in the intestines! This is a tremendous weight loss and health benefit and you don't have to jump through all kinds of oatbran hoops to get it - just gorge yourself on raw sex organs every morning! Not processed, boiled or stewed. Eat it raw!

Let me tell you another benefit that I personally recieved from augmenting my morning cycle with lots of luscious juicy fruits. I lead a very high stress life, and acquired the stomach problems you might anticipate from such an existence. I took reams of Rolaids, tons of Tagamet, and zimbles of Zantac. If you've got, or have had stomach problems, you know what I'm talking about. You've got a digestive tract that you've probably turned into chalk city in hopes of killing the pain before it kills you.

After being on this program several months, not only did I loose weight and feel energized, but MY stomach problems have completely disappeared for the first time since the twelfth grade (some ninety years ago). This benefit alone has made the diet worth it for me. You can not overestimate the wonderful feeling that comes from being really healthy, energetic and slim! The life giving, life sustaining, life building essence found only in sex organs has the power to transform your life when eaten daily. Believe it or not, when it comes to your body, sex organs make a huge difference, and without them, you're just not the same person!

I should make mention, of an initial effect that you're likely to incur as a result of eating fruit, particularly high water content fruit, every morning. You might get the feeling early on that you've eaten Loosner's Castor Oil Flakes, because of the state of your solid waste. In fact, you may see things you haven't seen in years. Don't be dismayed however (unless you happen to spend your mornings a considerable distance from the facilities created to expedite the process of elimination), because even though your reaction time may shrink initially, it's only a temporary phenomena. Once your body realizes that you're going to start helping it every morning, and gets most of the heavy cleaning out of the way, the large intestine will compensate because your body desperately needs the water!

However, the important thing to remember here, is that this is evidence that the five minute motor flush is working. As the body cleanses itself and grows accustomed to the fact that you're going to start working with it, rather than put up a big fight every day, your large intestine will adapt, and you'll be thankful that it did, believe me. You can look at it this way, any dietary regimen which can eliminate your need for suppositories is going to have it's supporters (and probably it's detractors. Can you imagine laxative companies coming out four square in favor of a diet that makes laxatives a thing of the past?). By the way, did you know that the way you say suppository in Italian is, "innuendo."

Finally, be sure you remember to follow through on your Anal Power Technique. Use all the time you need to anticipate improper dietary conduct (cheating) which may transpire later in the day, and correct those actions in your mind before they actually occur. This way you'll be presetting your response to temptation and it makes resisting a piece of cake!

The Importance of Becoming a Heavy Drinker

Before we get into the nature of, and the best way to eat heavy foods, I want to spend some time on the extent to which water contributes to weight loss. Water is one of the two things that we can't live too long without (the other is, as you might expect, television). Water does a number of vital things for us inside the body. Since the blood is about 90% plasma, which is almost entirely water, let's talk for a moment about the water in the system. As I mentioned earlier, not only does it provide for the transportation of various types of blood cells, it moves the vitamins, minerals, blood sugar, fat and hormones around the system. It also facilitates the washing of toxins out of the system with the help of your kidneys and your sweat glands.

Toxins in the blood can come from several sources. They can, as an example, be by-products of anaerobic combustion going on within the cells. This stuff is very toxic and must be carted away. In fact, one of these waste products (which will be discussed more completely in chapter 6), is the culprit that gives you the burn in your muscles when you work out. Part of getting in shape, is helping the body improve its ability to get rid of these toxins. Therefore, keeping hydrated, especially while you exercise, improves your body's ability to wash away this waste through your pee or your sweat. This will increase your endurance and your ability to sustain the fat burning process. This in turn reduces your warehoused inventory of fat even further.

Another source of toxins in the blood is what we eat. Without going into a long list of all the chemicals we eat in processed food and from pesticides used to control insects (and without making a value judgment as to how harmful these things might or might not be), it's safe to say that the sooner they get washed out of your system, the better. If it's allowed to be stored in your fat, (which is where it's usually put), liquidating fat cells from inventory at a later date can really increase the level of these toxins in your blood. While they may have gone into the fat gradually over a period of time, when you start dropping weight, they'll come out all at once. Nobody knows what effect they'll have while floating around in your system, waiting to be flushed away. So wash them away now!

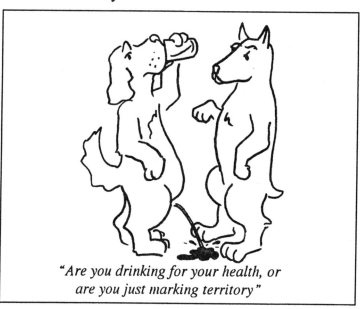

*"Are you drinking for your health, or
are you just marking territory"*

However, the most important benefits obtained from water in relation to weight loss (and this is why I advocate the drinking of eight, eight oz. glasses daily) are found in its ability to curb hunger and eliminate fat from the body. If you're hungry and drink a glass of water, what happens? Well it's like pouring a glass of water down a thirty foot tube.

It gets to the other end fairly quickly, which, I might add, is where the intestines are. When this glass of water starts to wash over the villi, digested particles of food that have been hanging around get taken up into a solution that the villi can instantly take advantage of, especially if you've already been cleaning them. The material is absorbed, the blood sugar goes up, the alarm goes off and you really don't feel like eating as much, or possibly even at all at that point.

The second way that water helps you to lose weight lies in the water soluble nature of some of the fatty acids in the body. Since the blood is virtually all water and since it transports everything in the system by its flow, everything transported within it must be dissolved one way or another in order to move within the system. This means that at any given point there is some, if not quite a bit, of fat dissolved and floating around with everything else in the blood. Fats that aren't water soluble are first encased in a protein shell by the liver, so that they too can float around in the body.

Your body knows that it needs approximately six quarts of liquid circulating at all times. When the level gets beyond the body's ability to cope, it signals the kidneys to filter and drain. What happens when you drink water is that not only do you flush the kidneys out and keep them healthy by helping to eliminate harmful deposits, but, as they filter the blood, some of those fatty acids (which would ultimately get stored in the adipose tissue and create more fat), get flushed out and eliminated with the other toxins. So you get rid of some fat without having to burn it. This is called weight loss without work!

It is also one of the reasons high water content fruits and vegetables help to make you skinny. They facilitate a process already in place to keep you trim. The reason fruits are so high in water content is tied up in the reason THE LIFEFORCE is there to such a great extent in the first place. A fertilized seed inside a container that is primarily filled with water is very similar in nature to a fertilized human egg inside a container that is filled primarily with water! Water is essential to life. It's the water found where THE LIFEFORCE is active, water that has within it those things that foster and accelerate the growth of life, that we want to fill ourselves with. The cosmic relationship between water, fruit, weight loss, and THE LIFEFORCE can not be overestimated!

These are some of the reasons (others will be highlighted in chapter 6) why drinking water, in addition to eating high water content fruits and vegetables, is of vital importance to the weight loss process. So here's what I want you to do, and you only have to be able to count to eight to do it: Start drinking eight glasses of water, not pop, not coffee, not tea or milk, but water, every day. If you want to drink those other things fine, but they don't count in your count to eight. Keep track of the number of glasses because you don't want to move down below five, for any reason whatsoever! You should definitely use the Anal Power Technique to visualize drinking eight glasses every day. See yourself at the end of the day finishing off your last glass and giving yourself a mental pat on the back. This will help to put your drinking on auto-pilot and pretty soon you'll have formed the habit.

One thing that I've found that makes drinking eight glasses of water easy is not drinking ice water. A big glass of ice water can sure taste great on a hot day... but we're not drinking to cool ourselves down. It's to gain health and loose fat. Drinking water that is either slightly warmer or a little cooler than the body won't shock the body the way ice water does and, as a consequence, goes down much easier.

If you love ice water and want to continue to drink it very cold and can drink eight very cold glasses of water a day, I think that's tremendous. But for those who don't want to shock themselves into submission eight times a day, don't hesitate to try it at various temperatures. You may find a temperature that enables you to think of water as a great thirst/hunger quencher and not some boring liquid used in the production of better drinks. Remember, count to eight!

At this point, let me mention a caveat about either drinking too much water and causing bloat, or drinking water while you're taking in substantial salt with your meals (and we're not talking either about your average drinker, or your average salt user here). We as Americans sometimes get it into our heads that anything worth doing is worth over doing. Sometimes we think if some is good, a great deal must be tremendous. This has been particularly noticeable in the drugs we take (both legal and illegal apparently) and the buffet dinners we go to. So don't feel compelled, when you see the weight falling off almost miraculously, to increase your daily intake from eight to fifteen glasses. Believe me, if you just continue to drink eight glasses a day (and it is important to keep it up) you'll loose a bunch of weight, no question about it!

The other caveat I mentioned is drinking water and eating a lot of salt with your meals. Salt is hygroscopic, which means that it takes in and retains water. The effect of this on your body is that because the water is held by the salt, it can't be expelled as easily. Too much liquid in the system over time can contribute to high blood pressure. That's why people with high blood pressure get put on low or no salt diets. So their system will more easily expel water and reduce the pressure on the pump and hoses.

Hence, if you have high blood pressure or high salt intake, be careful with overloading your system. Please note as well, however, that it takes a great deal to overload the system, and if ever there was an overload of anything in America, it's certainly not drinking water. So drink it every day and stay thin the American way, the same way the government goes through your tax money, by pissing it away.

So here's what you do every morning. Get up and have a big glass of sex organ juice, because this will start the washing process and charge you up with natural fructose right away. The next thing you want to do is gorge yourself on a high juice fruit, like melon. I love to down a big pile of cut up, de-seeded watermelon, honey dew, or muskmelon. Your sensor will tell you when you've eaten enough. Remember, whether it's peaches, grapes, any citrus fruit, plums, cherries, fresh pineapple, strawberries, or any other berry for that matter, you want juicy fruits, and they MUST be fresh.

Eating cooked sex organs is a waste of your time, as the life has been cooked out. In fact it's worth noting that once foods are elevated in temperature above 130 degrees, vitamins, proteins and other nutrients get destroyed. The longer your food stays above this temperature when it's being cooked, the less value there is nutritionally. That's why steaming and microwaving are better than boiling.

Putting the LIFEFORCE into your body every day is absolutely the key! As a matter of fact, I'll go so far as to say that the key to any good meal is that it's still alive when you begin to prepare it. Just as cut flowers continue to grow for days after they've been severed from the stem because the LIFEFORCE is still active within them, sex organs that have been picked only recently still contain most of the LIFEFORCE. But also like cut flowers, the fresher the better. During the day the goal is to eat as many foods as possible that still have an active LIFEFORCE. When you energize your body every day with this force, you will be filling yourself with life's essence and, by doing so, you can't help but notice the difference in your feeling of well-being. It's absolutely remarkable!

If you do happen to get hungry before lunch, drink a glass of water (have a glass of water even if you aren't hungry!), and have another piece of fruit. Don't eat anything but sex organs before lunch! If you're wondering whether you can eat it, just ask yourself, "is this a sex organ?" If it is, eat it raw. If it isn't, throw it back. The purpose of filling yourself with the LIFEFORCE is to fill yourself with its vivacious energy. Because we are what we eat, we must eat the right thing!

Do you know what happens to folks that forgo their big breakfast of meat and eggs, and have a big plate of sex organs? They don't feel like slugs, that's what. What's more important, they don't have to compensate for the digestive system's first call on energy by drinking a quart of coffee. You really can't appreciate just what you've been doing to yourself every morning until you decide to go back to the old load 'em up and drain 'em of energy breakfast, even as a change of pace. When you get this big lumpy mass in your gut and you just want to find a place to sleep, you realize, perhaps for the first time in your life, what eating to augment the natural digestive cycle does for your well being!

Healthy Combinations

Now that we've gotten breakfast out of the way, let's do lunch. Since lunch starts the next phase of the digestive cycle, we should delve into the other main category of foodstuffs, HEAVY FOODS. It's important to remember that while light foods contain the LIFEFORCE, heavy foods contain the weight. The reason is that they are made up primarily of densely packed tissue, usually processed and definitely dead! In this category we find all of the various types of meats and aquatics. It might be of value at this point to ask: Do you know the difference between meat and fish? Well, as any chef will tell you, you're not supposed to beat your fish...

Another group of consumables that should be placed in the Heavy Foods group is Starches. In this group we find all the various pastas, breads, rolls, muffins, donuts, crackers, cakes, cookies, pies and various tubers (roots) such as potatoes. From the things on this list you might ask yourself, "Are Starches bad?" Generally, I would answer no, unless they put too much in my shirts. Then I think, "If it's doing this to my shirts, what in the heck is it doing to my body? Is this why I feel stiff when I get out of bed in the morning, especially after eating heavy starch the night before?"

On the other hand, starches can have a great deal of value to you if you eat the right ones. Things like pastas and potatoes, for example, are complex carbohydrates, which are good for you when properly combined because they're easily turned into glycogen in the body, rather than fat. Glycogen (which is discussed extensively in Chapter 6) is a valuable energy source in the body, and a key component

of the fat burning process. So starches can be quite beneficial. The important point to remember about starches is that
it's great to eat the ones that are complex carbohydrates, and
less than best to eat the junky ones!

If you haven't guessed it already, one of the goals of this
dietary plan is to design your meals so that the digestive
system does a minimum of work. The best way to do this
is to properly combine your meals. Once you learn how to
do this (and believe me, it's a piece of cake!), there isn't
any need to set volume limits on yourself. You just stop
eating when you're no longer hungry. Ask yourself, "AM
I STILL HUNGRY?" If the answer is no, then for all
intents and purposes, you're done partner!

Before we discuss properly combining our foods, I'd like
to make an important point about the volume of our intake,
since we've managed to broach the subject. We live in
twentieth century America and, especially because we
want to drop weight, there isn't any need to clean up every
little morsel on you plate, ever again! We don't live in
Bangladesh. We live in the most prosperous, the most
bounteous country in the whole history of the world.
There's no need to feel a sense of guilt (imposed, no doubt,
in your youth by poverty stricken adults who were able, by
din of birth, to exercise great authority over your eating
habits) just because a misjudgment was made on the amount
of food needed on your plate at dinner.

There is no justification, that I'm aware of, for continuing to endure self inflicted angst because "your eyes were
bigger than your stomach." If you put too much food on your
plate and can't eat it all, save it. It makes absolutely no sense
to adhere to a completely arbitrary decision about how much
food you should eat. Especially if it's based on how much

food you can get on your plate!

Recent figures indicate that 62% of all Americans are considered overweight because we eat 72% more than the body's daily requirement. I believe this starts in childhood when parents decide arbitrarily what an adequate portion is, and then force their young to eat every last bit of food served or take the pipe. Bludgeoned with tales of starving children in other parts of the world, kids are forced by their parents to eat outrageous amounts of food, and for what? So they won't starve to death? If you're doing this to your children, CUT IT OUT IMMEDIATELY! Cramming food in your stomach until the last square inch is tightly packed serves no health or nutritional purpose whatsoever!

I come by this thinking rather easily because leftovers were never a sacrilege in our family when I was growing up. The most remarkable thing about my mother, in fact, was that for thirty years she continued to serve the family nothing but leftovers. The original meal was never found! There is however, a rumor floating around the family about a proposed dig in the old fridge.

Beyond that, I can tell you categorically that if you're done eating and there's still food on your plate, the starving people of the world will starve whether you eat it or not. If you've reached the age of majority, you're the boss, take charge! Believe me, there's nothing wrong with getting a little on the side once in a while! Don't turn your body into the local food bank. That's what you've got a fridge for!

If the ultimate goal of a dietary program is to teach you how to eat in a manner that not only leaves you slimmer, but allows your body to get all it needs nutritionally. A good dietary regimen shouldn't leave you feeling hungry, unsatisfied, tired or sluggish. In order to achieve these lofty dietary goals, I hope you would agree that it makes sense to know what to eat and when! It's just like the business world, where you should always know what to kiss and when!

Fortunately or unfortunately, depending on your perspective, the answer to the question of how to limit or even eliminate sluggishness after meals (assuming you're not suffering from coffee burn), feel satisfied, and continue to lose weight while you eat what ever you want, involves another key principle of the diet.

This is the principle of properly combining the things we eat at both lunch and dinner. Properly combining breakfast is irrelevant because all you should eat in any event is fruit!

The key principle of properly combining your meals is to SIMPLY REMEMBER THAT MEATS AND STARCHES SHOULD NEVER BE EATEN AT THE SAME MEAL! You can have all the meat you want, along with a generous helping of fresh or fresh frozen vegetables (remember the bulk of the meal should be living) or you can eat all the starches you want (again with a generous helping of vegetables), but never, never, never eat meats and starches together.

The question naturally arises, "Why shouldn't I eat meats and starches at the same meal?" The answer lies in the way these foods are digested in your stomach. Meats are digested with hydrochloric acid. This is very strong stuff. It has a pH of 1, which is about as strong as acids get (7 is neutral and 14 is about as caustic as it gets). On the other hand starches, because they're digested with enzymes that just happen to be alkali (alkali, caustic and base synonymously refer to liquids with pH values over 7). Something that is alkaline is the opposite of an acid.

Here's a question for you; What do you think happens when you mix an acid and a base? Well, what happens when you mix vinegar and baking soda? You get a lot of gas and foam, as each of the original ingredients ends up being neutralized by the other.

The bottom line, for all you bottom line folks, is that not very much work gets done, but you do get some gas for your trouble. What I didn't mention, but you should already know, is that it takes a hell of a lot of liquid energy from the blood stream for the glands in the stomach to produce the

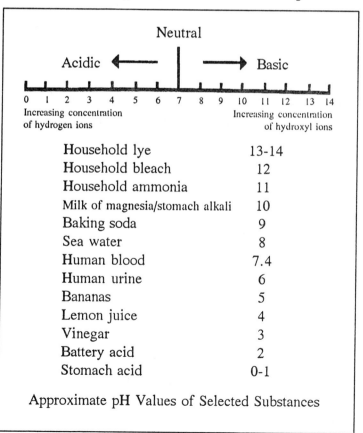

	pH
Household lye	13-14
Household bleach	12
Household ammonia	11
Milk of magnesia/stomach alkali	10
Baking soda	9
Sea water	8
Human blood	7.4
Human urine	6
Bananas	5
Lemon juice	4
Vinegar	3
Battery acid	2
Stomach acid	0-1

Approximate pH Values of Selected Substances

digestive juices doing all the work (As we've already discussed, draining the blood sugar for digestion triggers a feeling of tiredness). As the digestive juices become neutralized, a big tug of war starts between the opposing glands to see who's going to neutralize the other. This process ends up wasting a big chunk of your day's total energy allotment while you get tired and slug like.

This drawn out process of making more and more digestive juices reminds me of something my kids do. They turn on my flashlight and then put it back up on the shelf so it's on when we need it. It's great to know that you don't have to waste valuable time figuring out how to turn it on when the lights go out, but it sure wastes a bunch of energy in the mean time. Wouldn't you agree with me that it's a stupid waste of energy?

When we eat meats and starches together, we are either spitting into the wind or whizzing up a rope, I'm not sure which. The point is, if you avoid eating meats and starches together, you'll have quite a bit more energy, and your food will digest much quicker and easier. This will enable your system to extract more nutrients quicker. This leads your brain to signal your body to eat less!

Properly combining foods is the simplest thing, but it makes such a difference in your energy level. If you go out to eat and you've got a hankerin' for a piece of meat, do it. Remember, it's not what you're eating so much as it is what you're eating with what you're eating, this matters the most, particularly if most of the meal is living!

If you want to sit down and have a heavy food meal like a steak, several chickens or four or five fish, it's okay! Just have a salad and plenty of steamed vegetables. Forget the starches like bread, rolls, potatoes, and noodles unless you're going to forget the meats! This way there's no anxiety over calorie counting or worrying over what you can or can't have. It's very simple, it's one heavy food and all the vegetables you can eat! What could be simpler? Get in harmony with your body's processes and it will reward you by dramatically reducing inventories during your big spring clearance!

Planned Hunger

Finally, let's take a minute to talk about dinner or supper, whichever you have. I usually have supper, but every once in a while I have dinner. Like everything else in this crazy world, it just depends. But for our purposes it isn't going to matter that much, because the overriding factor is that the meal be properly combined and not be eaten after approximately seven to eight P.M.

The time that you have your last meal of the day matters for two reasons. The first is that you don't want to push the elimination phase of the digestive cycle too far into the next day. However, if you do shift work your schedule is going to be a little different than the average human being that goes to bed at night and gets up in the morning. Should this be the case, adjust your dietary regimen accordingly. But for everyone on the sun cycle, eating too late can and does push your duty further into the future, which can result in having to poop at all hours. We want to poop in the morning!

Another important consideration in deciding the best time to have your last meal of the day is your tendency to snack after hours. Normally every three to five hours, your body is going to ask you to refuel. If you eat at 4:30 or 5:00 in the afternoon and find that you need a snack about 10:00 (in order to get through the rest of your evening), you might want to consider having your last meal of the day an hour or two later. This way, you probably won't get hungry before you hit the sack.

It doesn't take a rocket scientist to figure out that eating a substantial snack before bed is not the best weight loss practice available. (Although rocket scientists are just as guilty of this as everyone else.) What you want to do, as part of your dietary life plan, is to pick and choose when you want to be hungry by pre-planning your hunger. What this means is to control your "hunger cycle." Due to the fact that we're creatures of habit, the point at which we feel hungry is, in all probability, pretty much the same every day.

So if you have a problem with being hungry and snacking at what seems like the same times during the day or night,

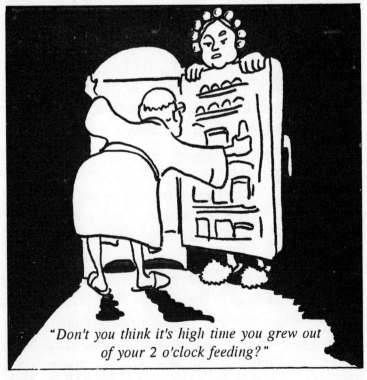

*"Don't you think it's high time you grew out
of your 2 o'clock feeding?"*

adjust your meal times to better fit your natural digestive rhythms. If you make the basic assumption that the body generally doesn't need to refuel for three to five hours after a meal, you can break up the time with several smaller meals, rather than one big one. As an example, instead of having a big dinner at 5:00 p.m. and ending up ravished by 10:00 p.m., have a good healthy snack about 4:00 p.m. and then dine at 7:00 p.m. Doing this often eliminates the need to eat at 10:00 p.m.

Another thing that helps you to avoid late night snacking is to go to bed just a little earlier. This way you can shave an hour off the night and add it to the morning, when you don't need to control your intake.

It is important, however, to stress that between meal snacks are not necessarily a bad thing. In fact they can be a good thing if used to postpone your hunger. What is important is that these snacks consist of complex carbohydrates. A very good case can be made for eating five or six small meals a day, which is much more efficient than a few big ones. A problem with having five or six small meals is of course that most working adults don't have the time to add several small meals to their daily regimen.

So for most people, a snack is more efficient. What you want a snack to do is shut off the hunger alarm. Never, never let yourself become overly hungry. One way to do this, as we've already discussed, is to drink a big glass of water. This works the best! Barring the availability of water, you could ignore the alarm, but that just isn't the American way. You will ultimately bring it under control with the Anal Power Technique, but that requires some effort, and hunger is right now. You could use will power and self denial, but if you lose, you might consider it a set back. Something clearly must be done, but what?

Well, since we already know that what shuts off the alarm the quickest is sugar (which is why all the things we tend to crave are made up primarily of sugar), we can do two things. If this craving is in the afternoon, there is nothing that will solve your problem quicker than a piece of sweet, sugary fruit. It kills the sugar urge on contact! If it's at night and you don't want to load up on food before you go to bed, there is still something you can do.

Fool your body! Go out and buy some sweet toothpaste, something like bubblegum flavored toothpaste, and brush your teeth! But don't just brush your teeth, brush your tongue and brush the roof of your mouth. What this does is to fill your mouth with sweet delight, and trick your tongue into telling your brain that some heavenly sweets are on their way! Additionally, by cleansing the mouth, you root out and eliminate little bits of food, left behind from your last meal, that are still digesting in the saliva and sending little ticklers to the tongue. If you don't clean them out, they will energize your taste buds and talk your brain into asking you for more good tasting food. So brush your teeth, the roof of your mouth and your tongue, to get them ready for the sex organs your going to eat in the morning.

If you shut your tongue off at the pass, your life will no longer be held hostage by your taste buds. If, when you get the urge to eat late at night, you thoroughly clean out your mouth and then drink a glass of water (remember, these are things that require no fighting, or conflict with yourself, about whether you should or shouldn't have the snack, there is absolutely no will power involved whatsoever!) you will totally eliminate the urge to eat for an hour or two. By the time this effect wares off you should be in bed.

This will set you free from the guilt, the weight, and all the other problems associated with late night eating. Instead of trying to force yourself not to do something and getting caught up in the swirl of disharmony created by your conscious mind (your will) pitting itself against your alarm system, you can choose not to play your tongue's silly little games. If you can escape being held hostage to your tongue, you'll be freer than you've ever been in your life. Free at last!

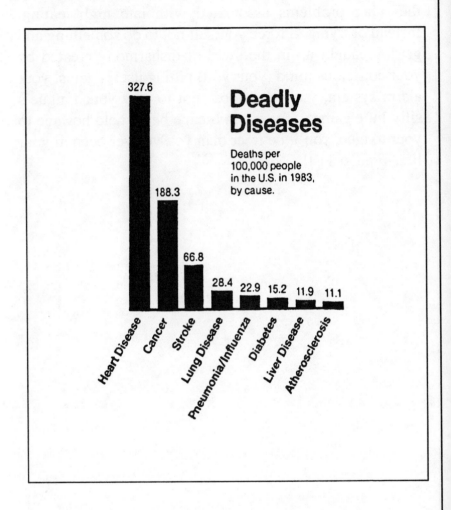

Deadly Diseases

Deaths per 100,000 people in the U.S. in 1983, by cause.

327.6 Heart Disease
188.3 Cancer
66.8 Stroke
28.4 Lung Disease
22.9 Pneumonia/Influenza
15.2 Diabetes
11.9 Liver Disease
11.1 Atherosclerosis

Chapter 4 -
THE IMPORTANCE OF MEAT IN YOUR DIET

Meat eating is pretty darned popular in this country, but then so is heart disease. The fact is, eating meat is a leading cause of statistics, which is something nobody wants to become. The scary thing is that the leading symptom found with heart disease is sudden death! I don't care how good your doctor is, that's one health problem he can't treat! There have been numerous research reports done in the last twenty years to indicate that there is a direct link between the ingestion of meat and heart disease. So, as your friend, I've got to talk about this with you.

Studies that have been international in scope clearly indicate that the level of heart disease in any given country is directly proportional to the per capita consumption of the flesh of animals, as is the level of cholesterol in the body. Non-meat eating cultures have much less cholesterol in their blood. The interesting thing is that when people from low heart disease countries come to our fair land, where the popularity of meat is at a peak, their incidence of heart disease rises to converge with ours, as their meat consumption increases.

Cholesterol, which is a tasteless, waxy, white powder, is

the big concern today in most medical circles, although I must say that the research on it's negative effects on the body is by no means complete. As an example, mammals such as the grizzly bear have outrageous levels by human standards, but almost no heart disease whatsoever. Beyond that, I can tell you that cholesterol is absolutely essential to life. Without it you would not be alive today. It is an essential component of cell membranes, and is at the base of key hormones in the body, such as the sex hormones. Try living without those!

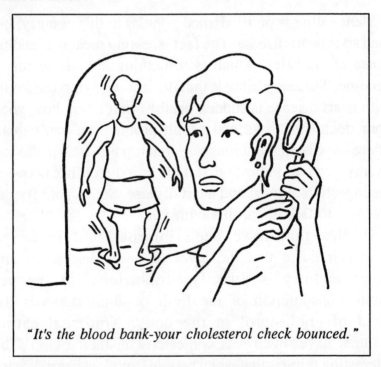

"It's the blood bank-your cholesterol check bounced."

But there is a substantial correlation between people that die prematurely of heart disease and high levels of low density lipoprotein cholesterol in the body. It's assumed that the waxy nature of cholesterol makes it easy to stick to the walls of veins and arteries, creating a build up of what is referred to as plaque. This plaque is responsible for most of the blockage that occurs in the vessels bringing oxygen to the heart muscle. Once a vessel is blocked, no oxygen gets to that part of the heart and it dies, never to be regenerated. The death of part of your heart muscle is very often terminal.

Everyone has to make their own decision about how much cholesterol affects your health. I just want you to remember two things. The first is that virtually all of the cholesterol you have in your body is not from eating cholesterol. Your liver makes it from fats in your system. The single biggest source of the fat that makes cholesterol so abundant in your system is unquestionably meat and the runner up is dairy products! The second thing I want you to remember is that when trying to decide how much cholesterol you can live with: a person who tries to be their own doctor, has a fool for a patient!

I should make it clear before we go any further, this isn't going to be another diatribe on the evils of meat eating. I love a tender, juicy slab of animal flesh seared on the grill as much as the next vegetarian (which I am not). Grilling it makes all the difference! If you can't have it smothered in all those carcinogenic by-products of combustion, why bother? There really isn't much like it, unless of course you like to grill your cigarettes. If that's the case, hey, don't worry about heart disease because you probably won't live long enough for heart disease to kill you.

I'm not going to pretend to you that meat is the scourge of the earth, because it can be a taste sensation! What we do have to be careful of however, is that today, the wide use of dangerous chemicals in the feed of all animals commercially slaughtered for food makes eating them even riskier than it used to be (when all we had to be concerned about was the inordinately high fat content choking the arteries of the heart, i.e. a lean piece of beef is still 50% fat).

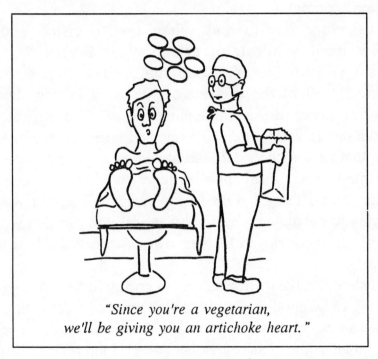

"Since you're a vegetarian,
we'll be giving you an artichoke heart."

One of the many problems that has lead Europeans to shun our beef is the extensive use of growth hormones. Keep in mind that cows can be legally fed anything that won't immediately poison us when we eat them. This can and does include everything from cement to sewage sludge pellets,which increase the weight of the animal. Its always a matter of, "How can we make the most money from the sale of this critter, in the shortest time possible?" In other words, what is the best way to prime the animal for sale.

Certainly growth hormones fall into this category. "If we

can make them bigger faster, we make more money- it's just that simple" said the rancher. But the one thing nobody can be certain of, is that if the meat you eat comes laced with growth hormones, will those hormones make you a bigger person for having had them? Everyone wants to be a big hearted guy or gal, but this probably isn't the way.

Does trying to lose weight while you're eating growth hormones sound just a little bit more difficult? Well, how about the fact that cows are fed materials to break down their tissue structure several days before they're slaughtered in order to tenderize their meat. Do you think it's going make you a stronger and more vital individual to eat meat laced with chemicals specifically designed to dissolve the flesh of the animal they happen to be in, in order to tenderize it.

Of course the USDA is firm in its belief that these things can have no effect on you, and I don't think they've ever been wrong. Can you think of a time the government swore up and down that something was safe and it turned out that they were about as wrong as one can get? You might just ask the people at Three Mile Island, or all the folks with cancerous tumers around Hanford, Washington, about government mistakes. I know one thing, they've certainly increased the demand for cancerous tumor research!

Poultry isn't exempt from the additive game. If anything, they're worse. Chickens are loaded with growth hormones that get them to full size in half the time it takes a chicken left to its own devices. They're fed arsenic to eliminate intestinal parasites and stimulate egg production. Do you find it interesting that every chicken born is injected with Turkey Herpes? That's right, every baby chick is injected with Turkey Herpes Virus, among other things, to prevent

Avian Merik's disease, a carcinoma in chickens. Does eating chicken flesh laced with Turkey Herpes virus make you want to gobble some. Probably only if it's barbecued, huh?

Is fish safe? Well, aside from the fact that fish farming is producing a fish heavily laidened with the very thing most people are trying to get away from when they eat fish in the first place, which is FAT, at some point you may want to ask yourself how much fish are affected by the polluted water they swim in. Fresh fish from the many polluted waters of our great nation, usually represents the "fresh catch of the day."

Interestingly, there is a group of concerned environmentalists that are now trying to get the State of Michigan to either ban or phase out 120 different industrial toxins dumped into the Great Lakes! Imagine if you can, 120 different poisons in the same glass of water! Unfortunately, this is probably not the worst case scenario for fish lovers.

The fish in the Great Lakes have been shown to have a number of things like mercury, lead, PCV's, PCB's, PCP's, and BMW's, (and a host of other things that don't sound any better), in their slimy little bodies. In fact many experts believe that the heavy metals accumulating in the bodies of Great Lakes fish account for the enormous weight of the salmon and lake trout taken from these lakes. I've heard fishermen tell stories of fish they caught no bigger than Blue Gills weighing over twenty five pounds because of all the lead and mercury in their bodies. Does this sound like a fish story? Well it is, but the point is quite definitely valid!

The east coast is <u>beyond</u> the worst case scenario. Places like Boston Harbor, have, for HUNDREDS of years been terminally polluted! (Was it Patrick Henry that said in effect,

"Give me liberty or give me death, but absolutely under no circumstances do I want you to give me any water from Boston Harbor!") Residents of the great State of Massachusetts have been dumping the worst kind of sludge into these very waters for several hundred years. I'm sure it's just an unfortunate coincidence that these are the waters where a very long list of the nations "Fresh catch of the Day" is extracted. Boston Scrod anyone?

The same can be said, however, for the Long Island Sound and the mighty Hudson. But let's not leave out Philadelphia and the rest of the faluvial cities along the east coast that have been nice enough to raise the continental shelf from a mole hill to a mountain. How fresh can the fresh catch be, when as far back as twenty five years ago the east coast, as a whole, was dumping FIFTY MILLION <u>TONS</u> OF WASTE A YEAR onto the continental shelf of the Atlantic Ocean.

This is of course in addition to the BILLIONS OF GALLONS a year of totally disgusting water, containing much more toxic waste than you could possibly imagine, flowing out of every major river entering either the Atlantic Ocean or the Gulf of Mexico.

With this in mind, we can't leave out our nation's largest river, the mighty Mississippi. The pollution, sewage, and toxic waste from literally hundreds and hundreds of cities is dumped into it every minute of every day! The nation's longest river, the Missouri, and the Illinois (which picks up toxic waste, pollution and sewage as it runs from Chicago down through a few hundred towns in Illinois), both dump everything they're carrying into the Mississippi around St. Louis, which is then carried south.

But if we mention these two, we can't leave out the Ohio, with all the waste it receives from the Allegheny and the

Monongahela Rivers at Pittsburg, where it forms. After it picks up all their waste, it meanders on down past big towns like Cincinnati, collecting toxic waste, before it also dumps the waste it's carrying into the Mighty Mississippi near St. Louis. These are only the very biggest rivers, there are literally hundreds of medium and small sized rivers doing the same thing along the way!

Kind of makes you wonder about that Gulf water quality doesn't it? Especially since it dumps right into the shrimp beds etc. of the Caribbean. We haven't even touched the rivers coming out of the great state of Texas, or Mexico, which doesn't even pretend to have pollution controls. Really makes you want to eat a bottom feeder doesn't it? Fresh oysters anyone?

The point of all this is not to convince you that if you eat the flesh of animals you're going to die tomorrow. Far from it, I'm sure you've got weeks. It is to say however, that eating the flesh of animals, and fish (which aren't inspected), and anything else fairly high up in the food chain can concentrate these toxins in a way that your body doesn't appreciate. It's the old story of one big fish eating a thousand little fish, which feed on this gunk. As the big fish digests the little fish the problem stays with the big fish until you eat the big fish and then his problems are over!

"But," you might say, "what do we do for protein if we shouldn't eat the flesh of animals or the many aquatics available to us?" It's interesting that all mammal life is ultimately derived from the plant world. We either eat plant life directly or eat those creatures which dine exclusively on materials from the plant world.

The question is: Why aren't the vegetarian animals that we eat, dying of protein deficiencies brought on by the lack of meat in their diet?

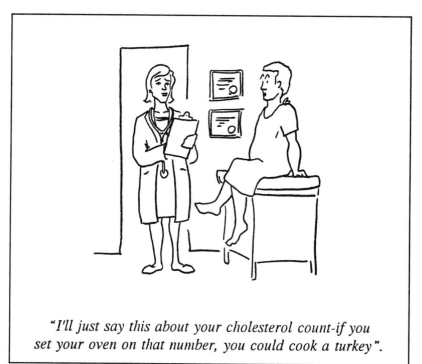

"I'll just say this about your cholesterol count-if you set your oven on that number, you could cook a turkey".

Isn't it interesting to you that many of the biggest, strongest animals in the world are all vegetarians. Look at such creatures as elephants, camels, oxen, water buffalo, buffalo, hippos, rhinos, horses, bulls, moose, giraffes, gorillas, and the Denver Broncos. We're puny next to these ferocious beasts. The gorilla, as an example, is three times as large and thirty times (that's right, thirty times) stronger than a human being, and he eats only sex organs when he can get them.

The myth about meat has more to do with the warrior / hunter ethic than it does about dietary necessity. Catching it and eating it was central to primal man's survival. Until the invention of the grocery store and the discovery of California, we had to work from dawn to setting sun just to get enough to survive. But because of the development of Capitalism, we have evolved into the kind, fun loving people we are today. Now we hardly ever say to ourselves while walking through the woods, "Oh look, there's a yummy little squirrel, let's eat it!"

Do you know how much protein you need daily according to the RDA requirements? (And this is with the usual safety factor built in.) People that are paid to look out for us say we need fifty six grams of protein a day, or less than two ounces. The average body only uses twenty three grams a day, or eight tenths of an ounce! Once this requirement is met, the body can't use any more (no matter how much you eat), so it's eliminated or turned into fat and stored. To replenish everything you need to remain completely healthy, you need about a pound and a half of protein a month!

Meats are far and away the hardest category of foods to digest. So heavy meat eaters are going to be quite a bit more tired after eating, as a rule, than non-meat eaters. For example, the lion, which everyone will agree is a major meat eater, only sleeps twenty hours a day! Gee, what a life, huh? While the gorilla, which, as we've mentioned, is a big fruit eater, sleeps about six hours a day.

See, the thing is this, meat has no fuel value, unless it's converted in a pinch by the liver to sugar and subsequently to fat, creating heavy waste that must be flushed away and eliminated. In addition, it has no fiber to aid its passing. So a heavy diet of meat tends to max out the digestive system, not only when it comes to breaking down the densely packed tissue, so the body can get at the amino acids and reassemble them into usable form, but because the intestinal tract has its work cut out for it just getting the stuff out the other end.

So if energy, vitality and vivaciousness are among the things we want in life, we need to eat things that contain these wonderful qualities. In order to exude all the wonderful qualities in our daily lives that are available to us, including sex appeal, it's singlely important to avoid making meat products the bulk of our meals. Let's concentrate instead on using Light Foods, which are the high fiber and high water content fruits, for breakfast and the life giving vegetables for lunch and dinner. Further, it's doubly important that we make sure to properly combine our meals (never mixing meats and starches) so that we don't squander a major percentage of our day's allotment of energy. In so doing, we are able to, as a consequence of this savings, redirect the energy toward projects and endeavors that are important to us. In this way we can get much more done in a single day than we used to, and appear to all the world as wonderful, exciting, energetic people that they really want to get to know!

Some people might think that it's a stretch to claim that simply by eating right you will become wonderful. However, it can be said that when we feel better, we act better. Quite simply, it's easier to be nice when you really feel good. This way of living will help to get you off the sugar roller coaster, something you may be on to a much greater extent than you realize. Some experts feel that this roller coaster ride produces behavior not unlike manic depression.

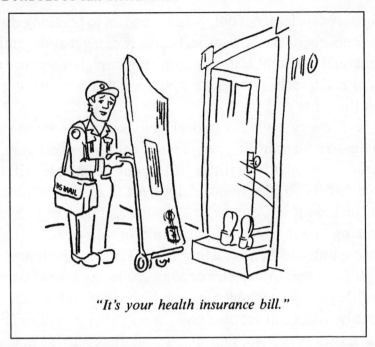

"It's your health insurance bill."

At first, you're really uplifted with the rush of the sugar coursing through your veins. But this big rush triggers an even bigger rush of insulin production which drains your blood sugar rather quickly. Then your mood drops through the floor, metaphorically speaking, when the sugar's all gone because there's nothing behind it to sustain the elevated state. It's like a big coffee burn! Remember, THE FABULOUS SEX ORGAN DIET is not a quick fix, but a way to live that will keep you charged up! Get excited about eating sex organs!

People are naturally drawn to people with energy. We love people who are exciting and alive without being hyperactive. We tend to admire people like this, probably because we're envious. My wife is such a person. She has the ability to go and go and go. She becomes relentless when honing in on a target. In fact, I often wish I had ten more just like her!

Conclusion

Reorganizing your daily intake, or your daily dietary regimen, to give yourself more energy, vitality, motivation and vivaciousness will make you attractive for the very reasons that you are attracted to, and admire other folks who seem to exude this life. It's an essential part of what comprises true desirability and sex appeal. Eating right will increase the very energy you need to get motivated to end, once and for all time, your weight problem. When you get sufficiently motivated to become relentless, I guarantee you that you will be wanted by the opposite sex! But whether you'll want them is the question. In the words of Gloria Steinham, "A woman without a man is like a fish without a bicycle!"

Finally, the sex appeal you develop won't be entirely centered on the lust of the flesh, but one that's much bigger than that which comes simply from being just another hard body! Believe me when I say that people love people who have the ability to get things done!

The question is; Can you get used to being loved that much?

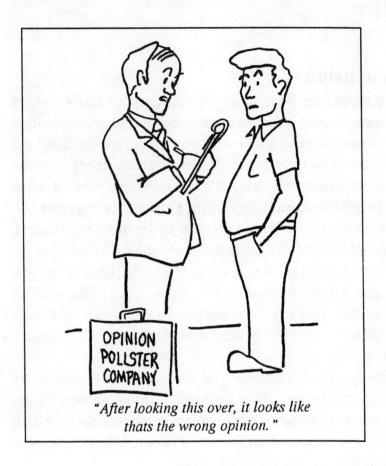

"After looking this over, it looks like thats the wrong opinion."

Chapter 5 -
GETTING FIT WITHOUT EXERCISE? BALDERDASH!

What is your attitude about exercise at this point? Do you think that exercise is for saps? Or maybe you've found that trying to get into shape is really hard and fairly boring? Have you found it difficult to sustain a workout program? If I can show you why it makes complete sense to do even a modest amount of exercise, would you be willing to try it again Sam? If What I was recommending was a piece of cake, would you do it then?

The fact of the matter is that regular exercise does so many good and enjoyable things, you would think that people would never stop, for fear of losing their benefits. It's hard to imagine how anyone could hold themselves back from something that provides so much natural appetite reduction, improves the salubriousness of sleep, strengthens one's bones, as it INCREASES one's strength, endurance, energy level, stamina, feeling of well-being, tone, shapeliness, and coordination.

Exercise raises the level of endorphins in the brain (a naturally occurring narcotic-like substance similar to opium), so that your level of peace, joy, and contentment goes up. It ENHANCES your sex appeal and your sexual enjoyment by creating stronger, more powerful orgasms. This in turn increases the demand for sexual experiences with your spouses and many loved ones. The ability to keep up with friends and/or business associates on outings and get-togethers will improve. It encourages the body to burn up the chemical by-products of stress and anxiety, which float freely in the blood-stream and have a tendency to make you feel like shit if they get half a chance. Finally, least we forget, it helps you to lose tons of weight by burning up fat on a greatly accelerated basis.

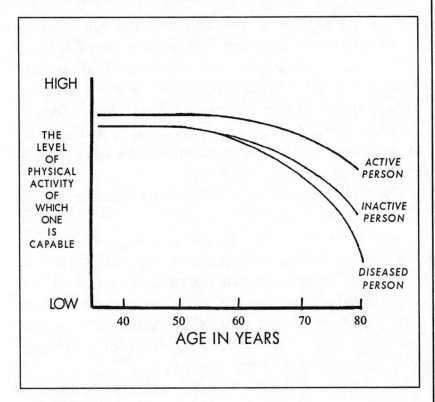

Curiously enough, for many people, simply hearing a description of the benefits is usually not enough to induce an action that is clearly in their own best interest. Having discussed at length why people often seem shackled to their past (and why the running start, discussed in Chapter 6, helps break these inertial bonds upon us by tying motivating emotions to that which helps us complete our goal), there's no need to reiterate that cogently written material here and now. Instead, I'm going to focus on why it's difficult to get around to beginning an exercise program, period.

The lack of desire is usually numero uno on the list of stoppers (why bother, who needs it, I've got too many more important things to do). A lack of motivation to do that which we KNOW is right, often stems from a low energy level just when the time comes to act. Being too tired and worn out to make the effort to correct the problem of being tired and worn out is easy to understand. Fortunately, with a running start it's not terribly difficult to overcome, if you want to that is.

Next, we find that because it might be hard and tiring, we really don't want the hassle. This is also easy to understand. Let's face it, things perceived as hard are easy to put on the back burner. At least until such time as our disgust with ourselves for not doing that which we intuitively feel to be the right thing, becomes greater than our fear of having to do something that might be hard. I call this DISGUST MOTIVATION. This type of motivation will temporarily give the project front burner attention, until we've acted on the situation long enough for the disgust to go away. Once the disgust goes, the project often becomes back burner material all over again, and our interest in following through dies shortly thereafter. Fortunately, what I'm advocating isn't hard in the least!

Another understandable reason is, of course, the fact that

it may be very little fun, and possibly boring in the beginning. When something is perceived as no fun, or boring (especially something you must do in your "spare" time), it definitely becomes back burner material unless there's an even more remote place to stick it (possibly where the sun don't shine?). Fortunately, once you get into the program, and start to feel tremendous (as the aforementioned benefits kick in), you will transcend fun and go right to pleasure!

In short, it's relatively easy to think of reasons why we can't - hell, I've got a million of 'em. What I hope to do with the remainder of this chapter, therefore, is to show you how doing a specific type of exercise over and over will help you to achieve your goals so much more quickly. You'll find the desire, the time, and the motivation, that is so essential to keeping it going.

Furthermore, it is my expectation that once you understand the nuts and bolts of the fat burning process, the whole reason WHY will suddenly make complete sense to you. When this happens, you'll do it because you can see for yourself that it's the way to go! Not because some know it all told you it was for your own good, but because you personally feel it merits your attention. We're told so many times during our lives that doing thus and so is for our own good, that often, no matter how well intended the advice, it usually ends up having the opposite effect, even if this source with which we take umbrage is probably right. So this time make up your own mind. Then, if it makes sense, swing into action!

Before we go on, I'd like to cover one more set of reasons why some people don't get with the plan. These are the excuses for which there are no excuse - ignorance, apathy, and stupidity. In talking with many of the failed dieters I've run into throughout history (people who've given up hope of ever getting thin) the story always sounds so familiar that I usually end up asking them if they truly know the difference between ignorance and apathy. They're usually so disappointed with their lives their response is almost always, "I don't know and I don't care!" Now isn't that one hell of an attitude?.

So let's forget ignorance and apathy, because those people don't read. Let's talk instead about stupidity, a malady common to both readers and non-readers alike. Leaving stupidity for the end of the list, I should add, is no indication of it's lack of stature as a problem. People who willfully flaunt their lack of concern for the facts about things that lead to heart disease (which is far and away the number one killer in the U.S.; if you have anything wrong with your body that you aren't aware of, statistically, you've probably got heart disease) are the very people who add substance to the mortality tables. Verily, verily I say unto thee, stupidity will be with you always, unfortunately. Fortunately, however, really stupid people have a short half-life, which keeps them from over populating. Unfortunately, their half-life isn't short enough to prevent them from ruining the earth with such things as pollution, toxic waste, nuclear waste and deforestation. Fortunatetly, you can make a difference!

I believe that it's important to point out (For the record), that because you had the good sense to read this book, you can't be in the aforementioned group. It's the other guys we have to worry about!

You know, now that I mention it, it's very interesting that God seems to have put definite limits on man's intelligence, but seems to have put absolutely no limits whatsoever on his stupidity, and frankly it's just not fair. You would think it would be the other way around, wouldn't you? Shouldn't a just God at least split it fifty/fifty? Wouldn't a loving God make it at least eighty/twenty in favor?

But I digress. More to the point is that inside every fat person is a skinny person with a lot of room. The process whereby we get the skinny person out from under the fat person takes strength, and that strength can be built by exercising good judgment in the use of one's muscles. In getting anything done, as you know, it helps to have the focus of a laser beam. But in order to get to the point where you even desire that kind of focus, the program has got to be palatable. Which means it's got to make sense, without appearing overwhelming. So here's what we're going to do; we're going to get you motivated, take the hardness out, give you the energy to get around to it before you disgust yourself any further, and formally banish ignorance, apathy, and stupidity forever from the face of the earth, Amen! Gee... No, GTE!

Before we get into the best way to exercise, let's take a quick look at fat formation, how it goes on and how it comes off. Fat is stored in three major places within the body. It's stored within all of your major muscles. It's stored around all the internal organs to a greater or lesser extent (depending on how big you are). Lastly, it's stored subcutaneously (which means under the skin), and this is the fat that makes you look fat. This last area is treated by the body's fat production center as kind of a last in, last out inventory storage situation. Which means it's the last place the body puts fat and the last place it goes to get it when it needs to burn fat for energy.

When we eat, no matter what we eat, it all falls into one of three main categories; health food, junk food, and my Mom's cookin'. Naturally, we can break these down into three smaller groups, generally referred to as carbohydrates, fats, and proteins. Each of these groups contains subgroups that can be broken down even further, naturally. Carbohydrates can be either simple or complex. Fats are either good or bad (unsaturated or saturated), depending on their effect on your health (fats in the blood are referred to as triglycerides).

It's interesting to note, that the only difference between fats and oils is that oils are liquid at room temperature, while fats remain solid. As an example, saturated fat is the white greasy substance that hardens in the frying pan after you cook a hamburger. The reason eating these saturated fats is detrimental is, that once they're in your system, they're going to do the same thing in your arteries that they do in the frying pan!

Finally, proteins are reduced to little Tinker Toys referred to as amino acids. All proteins are broken apart in the digestive system and reassembled into usable protein by the genes in the cells of the body. There are twenty three amino acids in total, fifteen of these the body can synthesize. The remaining eight the body must ingest to build a complete protein chain. Proteins are the building blocks of cell tissue, but once the building is done the remaining proteins are either eliminated as waste, or converted to fat and stored.

In a tight spot, protein can be converted to sugar, through a process called gluconeogenesis. For this reason, eating too much protein is not only pointless, but can actually be counter productive to your weight loss program. Protein is the hardest group to digest, so it uses the most energy going in, and often ends up as fat on the body instead of going out. The point is, eating too much protein is almost as detrimental as eating too much fat, and it definitely leads to extra work on your part, if you have to go back and burn it off!

CARBOHYDRATES

SIMPLE	COMPLEX
Concentrated	Diluted with lots of water and fiber
High calorie density	Low calorie density
Rapid breakdown and absorption - takes only a few minutes	Slow breakdown and absorption - takes hours to digest
Small particles	Large particles - broken down by mechanical action and digestive enzymes - fiber needs to be separated - cell walls must be broken down
Simple molecule - two sugars	Complex molecules - long chains, several thousand sugar molecules long
Split by salivary enzymes	Sugars split from ends of chain in intestines by enzymes from pancreas
Causes rapid rise in blood sugar to high levels	Gradual increase in blood sugar to appropriate levels
Requires large quantities of insulin	Requires small amounts of insulin
No vitamins or minerals	Lots of vitamins and minerals

Simple carbohydrates are sugars which after digestion end up as one particular sugar, glucose. This is the body's quickest source of energy and is also the food of the brain. Complex carbohydrates are starches that can be broken down into glucose or converted to glycogen, a polymer of glucose (a long chain of glucose molecules stuck together). Due to the fact that glycogen is a very efficient way to store sugar for later use (and is much better than having it turned into fat for storage), we truly want more glycogen production. Glycogen production is like putting food in the fridge for later use, rather than the freezer!

It's very important that we understand a little bit about glycogen, and how it contributes to fat incineration. Due to the fact that glycogen is a great source of energy for the muscles, the body stores it right next to the muscle cells, inside the muscles themselves. Think of it as great convenience store, kind of like a Seven Eleven for the muscles.

The problem with this, however, is if you don't burn it up, the body will convert it to fat, right where it stands. This produces what is called the marbling of the muscle. An example would be those little ripples of fat within the meat you buy at the store. It's what makes a good steak tender. As an example, the difference between round steak and a good Del Monico is that the muscle from which the round steak was cut was used all the time, and the muscle that provided the Del Monico was not.

One of the basic goals associated with losing weight is looking trim. But since the body will choose to use up the fat within the muscles before it starts on the fat under your skin, it'll be much harder to get to the point where you look thin if you don't unload your muscles first. That's why certain types of exercise are so important to the process of permanent weight loss. When you exercise in the right way, you literally ring out the fat from your muscles!

Once the muscle fat has been reduced, the body takes the fat in the blood (the triglycerides). As that level drops, the body starts taking fat from subcutaneously stored deposits in order to get the fat necessary for energy production. This process can take a while if your muscles are super flabby and your triglycerides are high. But regardless of how much time it takes, it'll always take less time if you burn it up aerobically than if you don't!

The body needs fat in order to burn glycogen for energy. The cell mixes fat with glucose (glycogen is converted back to glucose, as a precursor to the process) and oxygen to get a very high energy substance called Adenosine Triphosphate (ATP), which is finally burned for energy. This process eliminates a great deal of fat. The key to sustaining this process however, depends more than anything else, on the oxygen intake. Once your breathing becomes labored, limiting the oxygen being taken into the blood, and, as a consequence the oxygen available for making ATP, the cell switches to burning primarily protein. At this point, exercise stops doing what we want it to do. Primarily because we want it to burn mainly fat and glycogen for weight loss.

Here's the thing, our bodies produces energy for only three purposes. The first is for heat. The second is for the operation of our organs and gland secretion. The third is for locomotion. Heating the body takes a great deal of energy, and varies, with the season and how much we're actually outdoors. While the amount of energy the body burns for heat is pretty much out of our control, the amount of fat we carry affects the amount of energy we expend.

The reason is simple. Fat is the body's insulation, and just as when you insulate your house, your furnace burns less energy, the more fat you carry, the less the body needs to burn stored energy to stay warm. Gaining weight is like putting on a couple of sweaters. It makes the warming process more efficient and allows the body to store much more of what you eat. What all this means very simply, is that the fatter you get, the fatter you get, and the skinnier you get, the skinnier you get!

The second area of energy expenditure mentioned, transpires in the organs and glands. We have the least control over this process. The only effect we really want to have in this area is to conserve the energy consumed by digestion. As we've previously discussed, we want the digestive system to use much less, instead of more. Again, the reason is that digestion steals our quick energy and leaves us tired and sluggish. By avoiding sluggishness, our motivation level is much higher. When we "feel" motivated, we'll actually burn much more stored fat (which digestion doesn't burn). This is due primarily to the third reason the body burns energy, and the one we have the most control over, locomotion.

Locomotion refers to every single movement of the body. From the smallest and quickest, to the biggest and most pronounced, each requires an expenditure of energy. As we mentioned earlier in the book, weight loss is a simple matter of either taking in less than we currently burn up, or burning up more than we are taking in. Obviously, the fastest and easiest method of weight loss is some combination of the two. All we want is the fastest and the easiest, right?

Enter aerobic exercise. The first thing I want you to understand as we talk about aerobic exercise is that we're not necessarily talking about a class where a bunch of people jump around to music, although that certainly can be aerobic. What I want you to learn is, how you can judge when exercise is or isn't aerobic in nature. So that whether you decide to take an exercise class, ride an exercise bike, take walks, swim, put on some music and bounce some ounces in the privacy of your home or just do jumping jacks for twenty minutes, you'll know when you're aerobic and when you're not.

You will, as a consequence, be able to tailor a program to best suit your schedule. The goal of your exercise program should be to maximize the amount of fat incinerated without feeling so spent that you become useless. Exercise should make you feel wonderful (filled with endorphins), and if yours doesn't, we need to tweek it until it does! However, it is important to note, that getting your lungs in shape to handle the large influx of air needed to sustain the fat burning process is going to create some tiredness initially. But eventually, any tiredness that you feel at the conclusion of your workout will be momentary, BECAUSE THE SECRET TO BURNING FAT IS NOT TO DO IT HARDER, BUT TO DO IT LONGER!

Exercise falls into two main categories: Aerobic and Anaerobic (just as an aside, did you ever notice that there are two kinds of people. People who divide everything into two main groups, and those that don't). The difference in these categories, pure and simple, is whether the energy burn in the cell's combustion chamber is an oxygenated glycogen/glucose burn, or an un-oxygenated, primarily

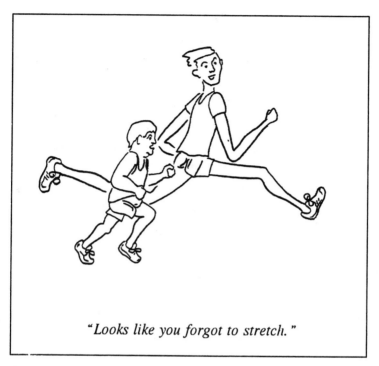

"Looks like you forgot to stretch."

protein burn, which produces toxic waste.

Essentially what we need to do to lose fat is to exercise aerobically. The key is to exercise at a level that allows us to breathe freely and easily, until we've passed what is referred to as the aerobic threshold. Once you're aerobic, you will remain aerobic until you either stop or run out of breath. The aerobic threshold is penetrated when you get your whole system involved in the work out. This is referred to as a systemic change, and the more different muscle systems you use, the quicker you'll pierce the threshold. That's why in aerobics classes they've got you moving everything you can possibly move, even your fingers, simultaneously, and continuously.

Fortunately, scientists have been able to determine

exactly when we break the barrier, and have related it to the speed at which the heart beats. The first thing you have to calculate is the rate at which your heart is maxed out. This is very easy, and assumes that you have no pre-existing heart problems that would alter what your heart is safely capable of. The way to find the average maximum heart rate for your age, is to subtract your age from 220.

Once you know your maximum heart rate, the point at which you break through the aerobic threshold is calculated as a percentage of that maximum. The first category we should look at is in the area of 50 to 60% of the maximum. This is the heart rate where so called "Low Impact" aerobics takes place. I should add here that "Low Impact" doesn't refer to the degree of effectiveness it has in terms of weight loss. It refers to the amount of stress placed on the body, and the joints in particular. I should further add that the idea isn't simply to achieve these heart rates but to sustain them, so that you prolong the fat burning process to the greatest extent possible.

At this heart rate (50 to 60%) you're burning primarily fat and some glycogen. This is the ideal area for "beginner worker outers," because it does everything to your body you want it to do, and yet it's not incredibly difficult to sustain for extended periods. It's great for people who have access to exercise bikes, particularly those that have arm movement as well as leg movement (remember, you want to move as many different muscles at the same time as possible).

The reason is that at this heart rate, you can go for extended periods (15 or 20 minutes, to over an hour) at a steady, moderate pace. REMEMBER, IT ISN'T HOW HARD YOU WORKOUT, IT'S HOW LONG, AND AT

WHAT HEART RATE. Obviously you'll want to work up to the extended periods if you can. The incentive is clearly there, because once you break the threshold you're guaranteed to be burning fat from then on, until you run completely out of breath, or stop. But please don't think that if you can't go an hour, it isn't worth it. If you only exercise aerobically 15 or 20 minutes a day, you will create the systemic changes that produce weight loss! Some is always better than none!

At 60% to 80% of your max rate, you are burning both fat and gylcogen together. This is where you get the maximum effect of aerobics on the body. Here the fat burning process starts to accelerate. Remember, in order to achieve permanent weight loss you have to eliminate the marbling from your muscles, and this is the best rate for that to happen. Subcutaneous fat can rise and fall and then rise again very quickly, so I'm not going to waste your time with a gimmick that may reduce your surface fat temporarily, but ultimately leave you worse off than before. The goal of this program is to make you permanently skinny! So ring out those muscles!

When your heart rate gets over 80% of max, your lung capacity has a very hard time keeping up with oxygen demand, and energy production rapidly goes anaerobic. This means that oxygen is lacking as a major component in the energy production process. Exercise can also go anaerobic at lower heart rates if you run out of breath. Preventing this from happening is a big part of getting into shape. It means pushing the capacity envelope of your lungs. This way, you can sustain moderate increases in your heart rate, because your lungs have gained the ability to keep up with the demand for oxygen. When this happens, your ability to burn the fat right off your body dramatically increases, because you can do it longer and longer without becoming totally spent!

As your aerobic program continues, tone will come as the marbling is reduced and the fat is wrung from the muscle. Tone is what produces shapeliness and the enticing curves we associate with the hot look. If you continue to exercise your muscles aerobically, they'll finally get taut without getting bigger. Muscle size comes from forcing muscles to do heavier and heavier work. What we're asking your muscles to do is not to necessarily work harder and harder, but longer and longer. This way they'll get tough and lean like round steak!

Now that you understand what aerobic exercise is, I want to take a moment and tell you about some of the physiological effects taking place within your body, and how these things help you to get you further along in your

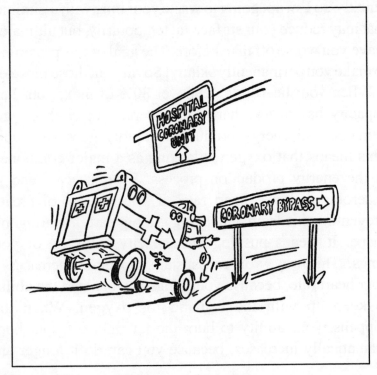

goal of getting skinny!

As you might immediately guess, aerobic exercise (AE) helps strengthen the heart. Like any muscle in the body that gets regular exercise, the heart will grow stronger, and it will get bigger. What this means to you is that as you strengthen your heart, you give yourself the capacity to prolong AE without strain, thus burning more and more fat at every sitting. As the heart gets bigger (which I should add is different from an enlarged heart, an enlarged heart is swollen) it's pumping capacity increases. As such, the heart doesn't have to beat as many times a minute to do its work. If, as an example, you drop your resting heart rate from 75 to 65 beats a minute, you will save 100,000 beats a week. What this means to you very simply is that just like any other pump, if it can operate it more efficiently at a lower speed, chances are, it will last much longer!

Once you get into full swing with the aerobic exercise program of your choosing, you can increase the blood flow through your muscles as much as thirty times the amount that goes through when they're resting. As a result of the work the muscles are doing, oxygen demands can increase as much as twenty times the resting amount, and heat production increases ten to twenty times the resting amount. What this should immediately indicate to you, is that there's a whole lot of burning going on when you exercise. Getting your lungs in shape to handle the dramatically increased flow of oxygen necessary really works in your favor!

Another point that should pop out at you is that with all the heat being produced, heat that if left unchecked will dramatically curtail or even kill the cells of the body, the importance of water to the aerobic process becomes evident.

Water is key to this process for two reasons. First, by simply being there to bathe the cells, and to provide water for sweat, it is instrumental in controlling heat. By keeping the heat under control, you can sustain the aerobic process that much longer. When you overheat, you will very quickly feel spent.

The second reason isn't as obvious, but it's still pretty important. When glycogen is created in the body, it takes three molecules of water for every one molecule of glucose, to make one molecule of glycogen. What this means to you is that if there is surplus water available to the body during the glycogen production process, the body will make substantially more glycogen than if it can't get the water. Here, the benefit to you is that because the alternative to glycogen production is fat production (and once it's fat, it's fat forever until it's burned), your body will make less fat and more glycogen. This in turn serves to burn even more fat when the glycogen is oxidized! SO DRINK YOUR WATER!

Now that it's plain to you why AE will go a long way toward furthering your heart felt aspirations, let's take a look at anaerobic exercise (AAE), and examine it's drawbacks as a method of weight control. First, let's understand exactly what we're referring to when we talk about the dreaded AAE. At the cell level it occurs when material is metabolized for energy production without adequate oxygen available to support the burn. It's like the burn you get from the welder's torch when the oxygen knob is turned off. The flame is of poor quality and you get a sooty, messy burn that has to be cleaned up or the cell will die!

Exercises requiring brief spurts of intense effort (weight lifting would be one example) are anaerobic. When the speed of the heart can't increase fast enough to get the added oxygen necessary to the cells to produce ATP, the body starts burning protein, which doesn't require as much oxygen to burn. It's kind of like the old story of the guy who has to burn the family furniture to heat the house because the coal man forgot to deliver the coal and everybody's freezing. Naturally the guy would like to save his furniture for its express purpose, but some things take precedence, as energy production will do over cell repair. For this reason, you definitely want to keep the coal man coming!

Another problem with AAE is that water begins to be lost at an accelerated rate as the body tries to rid itself of the soot. As you know, this soot is completely toxic, although not immediately deadly (It would kill you, however, if the body didn't have a method in place to eliminate it. This is why kidney failure is fatal!). These toxins include but are not limited to, such things as full strength ammonia, urea or uric acid (the cause of gout when the body starts to store it in the joints to get rid of it when it piles up), and lactic acid. Lactic acid is the material that causes the pain in your muscles when you refer to them as being "over worked."

While aerobic energy production creates a burn that releases pure water back into the cell, bathing the combustion process, and facilitating processes within the cell that enables the burn to continue (as well as freeing up water for heat control), AAE just makes a big mess. To wash the toxins away, the body must use the water it might otherwise use to bathe and cool the combustion process. This in turn, forces the excretion of valuable electrolytes along with the toxins, via the sweat, and kidney filtering. (Electrolyte depletion is the primary reason for muscle cramping, which of course is a real pain.)

Electrolytes that are caught up in the flush include: Potassium, which helps control muscle temperature, blood flow, and nerve conduction; calcium, which, in addition to improving bone strength, is essential for muscle control; and magnesium, which helps regulate muscle contraction and the conversion of carbohydrates to energy. Sodium, which is obtained primarily from sodium chloride (table salt), is also lost. But it's not critical that we concern ourselves with losing it, because salt is the most abundant mineral in the body. We only need 1/2 a gram per day (500 miligrams) and that is easily gotten from the food we eat, without reaching for the salt shaker.

One of the big problems with salt is that it holds water in the body. The reason is that the body must dilute the salt down to the point where the water plus the salt creates a solution that is balanced with the rest of the body's salt to water ratio, so you don't die of salt poisoning. Water will automatically rush right to the stomach, to balance any ingestion of salt. That's why taking salt tablets when you work out is the worst thing you can do for muscle performance and fat reduction, because the cells need the water much more than the stomach does!

In summing up anaerobic energy production we can say that once anaerobic activity starts, the body begins to struggle with energy production. The internal cell temperatures rise to the point where cell processes begin shutting down, toxins start building up, while electrolytes become depleted, and the cells finally become dehydrated. At this point, the whole energy production process breaks down, allowing pain and fatigue to set in.

As you should easily understand at this point, water is extremely important to weight loss. But here's something even more important to remember: The feeling of thirst will not arrive in time to head off the breakdown of the process of fat combustion at the cell level, due to cell dehydration! Drinking eight glasses of water a day has nothing to do with thirst, it's for maximum fat incineration, glycogen production, heat control, and toxic waste removal cell by cell! If you wait until you feel thirsty before you drink water, you'll lose the battle!

You now see before you the essence of both aerobic and

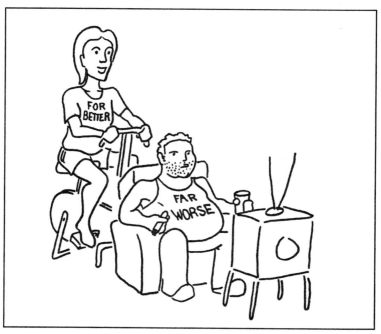

anaerobic exercise. From this information, it should be clear to you why all the sensible weight loss experts advocate regular aerobic exercise as part of a successful weight loss program. If you don't burn up the collected fat within the muscles first, you have to eat a heck of a lot less in order to get the same net effect. As we've already discussed, starving yourself never works beyond the temporary, because you're so miserable that falling back into the old comfort zone seems almost a welcome relief!

This is why it's very important to start out slow and work up to a full fledged workout. When you start out slow you get the thought going through your mind that what you're doing is too easy and you can do more. The feeling of longing for more is much better than feeling that you're in over your head, and you wish you could quit. What you want to do is increase your effort layer upon layer, week by week, until you get to the point where you're really challenged. At this point you will start to push the aerobic envelope. As you do, fat combustion will accelerate. Then, just keep the envelope expanding a little at a time until pretty soon that little envelope you started with is now a great big mail bag!

The last thing you want to do is try to take on the world the very first day, go anaerobic almost immediately into the workout, and produce needless pain and suffering. Pain and suffering might easily serve to discourage you and get you off the track before you get a chance to feel the tremendous benefits of what you're doing! Take the time during the "mental running start" period to plan the layers ahead of time. You might look into classes, you might get the old bike tuned up, or even acquire some sort of exercise machine to break the aerobic threshold. This way, when you hit the successive layers you've planned, it'll make you feel like you're really doing it, and that progress is being made on all fronts!

<u>REMEMBER, IT'S NOT HOW HARD YOU WORK OUT, BUT HOW LONG AND AT WHAT HEART RATE</u>. Further, the more different muscle groups you use, the greater the number of independent signals being sent from different locations in the body to the brain, demanding an increase in the supply of blood and oxygen. The greater the number of signals, the sooner your body kicks into gear and blasts through the aerobic threshold, thereby accelerating the fat burning process!

Now you understand the process, and can easily explain to your friends and countrymen why exercise has been given a bum wrap. You clearly do not need to knock yourself out to be successful. You only need to be relentless. If you couple THE FABULOUS SEX ORGAN DIET with a palatable aerobic workout program, you will find the results absolutely staggering!

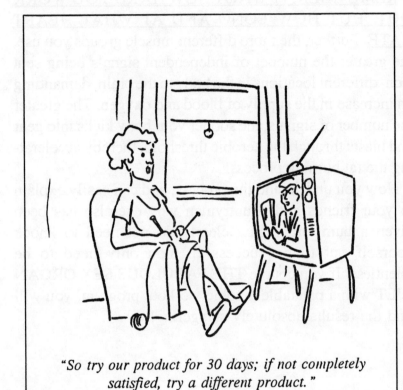

*"So try our product for 30 days; if not completely
satisfied, try a different product."*

Chapter 6 -
D-DAY: LAUNCHING THE PROGRAM

Ah, to capture the beginners spirit! Great thinkers throughout the ages have commented upon the fact that something well begun is half done. Starting properly is so important that I decided to dedicate an entire chapter to the best way of getting started. What I hope to accomplish with this segment is to get you started with a process that takes you off the drawing board and into self actualization. In order to maximize your chance for complete success, I want to give you every edge. As a further aid in this transition, I have included my own beginnings on this new way of life, which will be found in the next chapter.

Just what is the beginner's spirit, and how do we capture and use it to our advantage? Simply put, it is the excitement and enthusiasm we feel at the beginning of a project we really want to take on and complete. We exude a dynamic, motivating energy as beginners when we face a task we're excited about. It wells up within us and gives us impetus. When we bring this energy to bear on a single project, using the focus of a laser beam, we get a push that takes us well into the project before we even begin to be subject to the little stumbling blocks that start to suck the gumption out of us and rob us of some of our vital energy and enthusiasm for the task.

A force that the beginner's spirit helps us to overcome is the inertial resistance that has stalled many a well intentioned project. We all remember inertia from high school science class, right? It's one of the most cosmic laws of the universe. It applies as much to the actions of humans as it does to inanimate matter. The law states very clearly that an object at rest tends to stay at rest, and an object in motion tends to stay in motion. A corollary to this law states basically that it takes a great deal more energy to get a resting body in motion, than it does to keep it in motion at the last (most recent) speed attained.

You can see this with your car. It takes a great deal more gas to get the car from zero to sixty than it does to keep it at sixty. That's why stop and go driving consumes a great deal more gas than highway driving. It's the reason the first stage of a rocket is so much bigger than the later stages. It's the same for the powerful locomotives pulling a long train. They always put extra engines on to get that mother started, and then, after the train is up to speed, they throttle the extras down. It just takes more energy to get going than to keep going. Once moving, the only force that needs to be expended to keep moving is that force necessary to overcome friction.

The other side of this law is just as important for our purposes. The flip side of this law, which deals with objects already in motion, states that it's much harder to stop an object that has built up a powerful momental force than it is to stop something barely moving (very little momental force). It's quite simple actually; once an object has momentum, it is much more difficult to stop. In addition, the more momentum created, the farther the object will carry before needing another push. We see this in everything from sledding down hill to victories in sporting events. How often have we seen the underdog gather momentum and come from behind to win? Momentum is the reason it takes miles and miles of track to stop a fully loaded train. It's the reason ships must throttle back long before getting to the breakwater outside the harbor. This law is absolute and affects everything on earth! The point is this: you want it working for you, not against you!

The big question then becomes: How do we develop a strong beginner's spirit, a powerful motive force that will enable us to bust through all the roadblocks and barriers standing in the way of our stated objective? My feeling, and one that has been corroborated by other motivational experts, is to get a running start! High Jumpers don't stand at the bar, over seven feet from the ground, and try to pop over. Pole Vaulters don't do it, Long Jumpers don't do it, and neither should you.

When a football player has to muscle his way through the line, he doesn't start at the line and begin to push. He starts running as hard as he can from five yards back. In fact, simple common sense should tell you that if you must jump a crevice, you don't stand on the edge and leap, you get a running start so that the momentum, coupled with the spring of the jump, will get you to the other side. It will always be harder to accomplish what you need to get done, if you just stand at the edge and leap. So here's what you do, here's how you get your running start!

Set a target date, anywhere from one to three weeks into the future, and plan on actually starting the program that day. It's the same thing you might employ if, for example, it's Monday and you've got something planned for Saturday that has you so excited, you just can't stop thinking about it. You're thinking about how much fun you're going to have, and how wonderful the whole thing is going to turn out. The value of this approach is that it gives you time to build a rock solid personal commitment to actually following through.

As we mentioned earlier in the book, if you're going to change what are essentially unproductive habits, habits that, for whatever reason, are no longer useful to you, and substitute better ones, you're going to have to get serious. Playing at it for a week or so will only lead to further dejection and more misery about a condition you've probably come to loathe. That's why I want you to start planning ahead with your mind using words, pictures and, particularly, emotions. Make them the very strongest emotions you can possibly muster (as you obviously already know, simple logic has no motivating power whatsoever, for anyone other than Spock) this way you'll be so charged up by game time that your running start will enable you to soar clear over the barricade and get fifty yards down the field before the opposition knows you've even got the ball.

I want you to look at getting started on the program as you would view going on a trip you've always wanted to take. You've spent a great deal of time dreaming about this trip your entire life, and in just a few short weeks you're getting on the airplane! But like any trip of several weeks or more, the preparation has to be done so that you'll have a blast. The time spent dreaming and planning heightens the build up of anticipation, and this is what gives you your running start! If you were going on a hiking trip, you would go shopping for equipment, read about the country you're going to traverse, look over the maps available to study your route, and think about all the fun you're going to have when you get there. These are the things that get you pumped.

If you were going to a beautiful tropical paradise you'd go shopping for new outfits. You'd read a little bit about the place and all the things to do there. You'd start planning the various details of the trip, such as how and when you're going to arrive, where you're going to stay and how much all this is likely to cost, (even if money is no object). For the trip of a lifetime, you'd be psyched and ready!

This is how one develops the beginners spirit! It's what's going on in your head while you're doing the preparation, and experiencing the anticipation that gets you totally psyched. Once again, it comes down to the most fundamental of all the principles concerning preparation, CONSTANTLY VISUALIZING every aspect of the way you WANT things to go! See in your mind: starting the program, being on it, following through with it and being pleased with yourself. See yourself successfully resisting improper conduct, and getting the results that are unquestionably available to you. There is no limit to all that you can visualize in conjunction with beginning and continuing this program until you've achieved complete success! The key is to get so pumped up (and I mean this in the sense of building relentless determination, not simply getting wired) about doing this that once you jump on the sled and start downhill, the momentum just gets stronger and stronger as you pick up speed. There is a tremendous feeling of exhilaration tied to the excitement of actually becoming that train moving relentlessly down the track to the destination!

Every time you think about it, tell yourself you're going to do it, and SEE it happen! You should tell yourself things like, "I'm going to do it, I'm going to do it, damnit I AM going to do it on the date I've set!" Direct every free thought to it. In addition, direct as much conversation as possible to it, so that you put yourself on the hook. Start living, breathing, and feeling the start and follow through of your new dietary regimen. Do it to the point where what you want becomes so internalized, and your system is so totally absorbed in the idea, that your TIC and your auto-pilot will carry you through -- no matter how heavy the burden, or how many times things have fallen apart for you in the past!

Developing this single mindedness and relentless deter-mination ahead of time will produce so much pent up power that when you start, you will definitely hit the ground running! This is exactly what the coalition force leaders had the troops do in Saudi Arabia- for six full months-before they actually got the chance to engage the enemy. When they were finally uncaged, unchained and pointed in the right direction, they were so awesome and performed so well that they literally astounded the world. You can easily put this same motive force behind getting to your objective. Thoughts of compromise and failure are taken out and shot!

There need be no thought of anything but succeeding, absolutely and utterly. If unproductive thoughts do creep into the visualization process, don't give them any energy whatsoever. Simply replace them with visualizations of the way you want things to go. If you remember nothing else, please keep this extraordinary fact in mind every single moment of every single day for the rest of your life, because it's that important. This completely dominant law of nature is simply: THAT WE BECOME WHAT WE CON-STANTLY THINK ABOUT!

There is no law more fundamentally important to your future life than this! Your mind actively pursues and works to bring about (on both the conscious and subconscious levels), that which you think about. The danger in this is that it works just as hard to bring about that which we fear, if we're always thinking about that fear. By visualizing the outcome of a fear that might be gripping you, you are setting your TIC and your auto-pilot to work on bringing about the very thing you loath to happen!

For this reason, it's vitally important not to give your fears the time of day! In your life, you cannot afford to set in motion counter-productive forces which will wreck havoc with your mental state, preventing you from focusing on what you really want! What you think about every chance you get will become stronger and stronger as you continually visualize it as an outcome.

So if you're caught up in fear motivated thinking, it becomes the worse kind of self-sabotage, not only because are you continually shooting yourself in the foot, but you're actually encouraging the bleeding. This loss of blood makes your whole body weak, and everything in life much more difficult. At the very least, it increases the friction you feel while going through life, and as you remember, friction is the enemy of momentum. If you don't cut it out, you will hobble around until you stumble and fall right into the midst of your worst fears, just as you visualized it a thousand times before!

This is why, when you get started by having previously

tied strong, positive emotions and visualizations to your objective, you become much, much harder to stop! It takes your mental laser beam off your foot and puts it on the target. The reason for practicing in your mind every single moment of every single day is that you've got a lot of old tapes that must be erased. As these are erased and replaced with new ones, they will have the effect of dramatically reducing the friction that eats away at your momentum and slows you down. Changing those old movies to new ones is the difference between sliding on concrete and sliding on ice.

So when a negative thought pops into your head, cross it out, push it off the stage, and replace it with the very best thought possible in terms of your goal. This will help you to become relentless, single minded, and determined to do whatever it takes to succeed. By tying powerful emotions to the idea of starting and sticking to your new dietary game plan, through the use of visualization and self-talk, you'll have all the processes of change aligned in your favor; and as you have to know, that's a pretty powerful armada sailing off to victory, fighting in the Gulf between where you are and where you want to be!

Starting the program the minute you finish the book might work, and you might even be incredibly successful, since eating sex organs every day is a powerful way to lose weight. But, just as George Bush waited until all the troops were ready to march before having an Iraq-attack, taking some time beforehand to lay the ground work and plan the invasion gives you a better shot at total victory! Think of it this way, habits, which start as thin cob webs, grow to thick cables that will either be your lifeline (if they're constructive) or binding shackles (if they're self-defeating). What you're going to do is to start sawing on the cables for awhile before you start trying to break them!

By picking a target date and readying your mind, body and soul, you'll be doing exactly what the allies did to get ready for the invasion of Normandy. When you marshal all your resources ahead of time, not only are you ready, willing, and able to go at it, but you become a cruise missile, a proverbial Tomahawk aimed directly at the target, rather than a mortar shell lobbed into an area. So build your momentum by getting a running start!

Practicing in your mind is the only way to reset your TIC, and is the method by which you replace old habits with new habits. Practicing in your mind not only saves time and wasted effort, it's the extra edge that top professionals in every field employ to perfect their performance ahead of time.

A study was done some time ago by a fellow named Maxwell Maltz, M.D. who wrote, <u>Psycho Cybernetics</u>. The results were quite revealing. In this study, he took a basketball team and divided it into three groups. The idea was to determine the best way to improve the team's free throw shooting. Group one shot on the first day, didn't practice at all during the next twenty one days. They functioned as the control group. They were tested again after twenty one days, and as you might expect, there was no improvement.

The second group was instructed, after being initially tested, to practice twenty minutes every day for the entire period of the test. The third group, after being tested, was told to sit for twenty minutes every day in a quiet place and practice in their minds. They were to be very graphic in their visualizations -- seeing everything from the placement of their feet on the free throw line to how they held the ball.

The players who actually went out on the court and shot the free throws every day for twenty one days, twenty minutes a day, improved. Their performance was up 24%. However, the incredible thing about the test, was the score of the third group, the one that didn't put their hands on a basketball. They were up 23%. The fact that all the practice took place in the mind tells you just how powerful this technique can be!

It should be completely clear to you at this point that the idea of practicing the launch and follow through ahead of time in your mind greatly improves your chance of success. That's why the NASA astronauts were required to practice every single step involved in going to the moon, over and over, in their minds. They took something that nobody had ever done before, and made it so habitual, so routine, they didn't even have to think about what to do when the time came to actually do it. When they went to the moon for real, it was easy because each response had long ago become automatic.

One of the things that both the basketball players and the astronauts had in common was that they took time EVERY DAY to repetitively review a sequence of anticipated actions or events they knew they would eventually be required to repeat in actuality. That's why the ANAL POWER TECHNIQUE is so important. In the midst of all the hustle and bustle of your schedule, you have to take time out of your schedule, no matter how busy you are, to take a poop. It's the perfect opportunity to tune out the world, and tune in your future actions.

By doing this, you will not only have a dramatic impact on your conduct over time, but you will be greatly helped in your effort to sustain your initial momentum. You will set in place, patterns of conduct, relative to a particular event, in your mind before hand. When the event actually transpires, the mind will reference the information already stored about the event. The mind will then guide the body in reproducing, in reality, the prerehearsed, prerecorded patterns. Does this sound too incredible to be true?

Does it sound like something others can do but you can not? Would it surprise you to learn that this is exactly what your mind does when you're driving and become lost in thought. Your mind has been trained by your repetitive actions to drive in a certain manner, whether you're paying attention or not (as long as you continue to sit there with your eyes open, looking ahead of course).

I'm sure you've often found yourself breaking without giving it the slightest thought. Snapping out of your daydream, you find that the guy ahead of you slowed down and it was a good thing you put on the breaks when you did or you'd be eating steering wheel. But at the instant your mind acted to save you, you didn't have to be rigidly focused on the car ahead, you had already preprogrammed your mind to do exactly what you wanted done. When the time came to act you didn't have to think, because thinking wasn't required. The actions were automatic. All that was required was for the brain to access the prerecorded response from storage and execute the response. No thinking on the conscious level was involved.

This programmed response mechanism also controls your eating habits. That's why you must reset it. If you don't, much of your eating will continue on an automatic pilot setting that's still relying on old outmoded tapes, tapes that contain programmed responses that run counter to your new wants and desires!

Conclusion

I have just laid out for you the central ideas behind why setting up a D-DAY makes more sense than just lunging at the target. When you're emotionally committed, and primed for success (your TIC pre-set and your auto-pilot ready to steer), you will have a tremendous running start. Once you've crashed through though, be sure to continue to use your new visualization process as often as you can. This will help to reduce the friction that zaps motivation and keep you honing in on that target you've set!

Remember, a body in motion tends to stay in motion.

All you need to do, to keep going, is to practice in your mind every day what you want to achieve in actuality. That way, you'll be doing just what the coalition forces did while getting ready to attack-Iraq, and your chance of success will be overwhelming. You will find yourself blowing past hurdles, which used to cause you to stumble, before you even think about them. THE BEAUTY OF THIS IS THAT WILL POWER IS ABSOLUTELY IRRELEVANT TO THE PROCESS! Whether you have a strong will, a weak will, or no will at all, it really doesn't matter. The reason is; the will is a tool of your conscious mind. We use our will to try to force ourselves to fall in line, behind the wishes of the conscious mind. It's a tool used to force part of you to do what the other part wants.

If your will is good at the application of force, and is accustomed to having it's own way, you probably feel like you have a great deal of will power. If force doesn't work on you or your conscious mind can't seem to turn the right screws when it wants action, you might feel like you have little or no will power. But regardless of the level of will power you think you have, it really doesn't matter!

If you feel that you've been failing in the weight loss department because you don't have any will power, then you're going to be PERSONALLY EXCITED! Because we're completely cutting you out of the will. The only thing we're asking your conscious mind to do INITIALLY is to feed the emotionally charged visualizations you're generating into your subconscious; and since that's really a no brainer... You don't have to force yourself to lose weight any more!

You'll be much better off, and more effective, letting the same mechanism that does your driving when you mentally wander off, handle the hurdles. Just make sure that, like the astronauts, you take the time every day to do the graphic visualizations that will reset your TIC. Put as much emotion and feeling into these visualizations as you can muster. Do them night and day, day and night, and every moment in between. Every time the subject enters your mind before D-DAY use it as an opportunity, and once you're launched, keep it up! That way you'll be invincible!

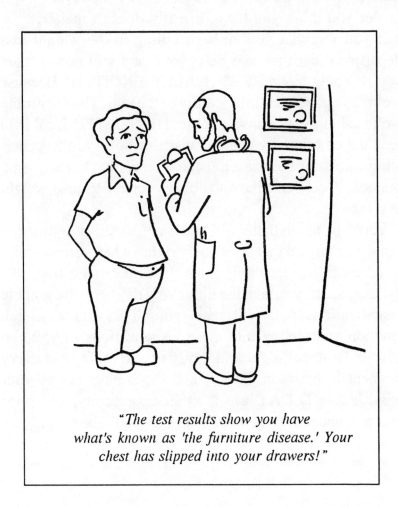

*"The test results show you have
what's known as 'the furniture disease.' Your
chest has slipped into your drawers!"*

Chapter 7 -

THIRTY DAYS HATH APRIL, JUNE, AND THE FABULOUS SEX ORGAN DIET!

As part of trying to develop a diet that all Americans could welcome with open arms, I thought perhaps that if I could get it to work on me, it would work on anybody. Similarly, I felt strongly that coming out with dietary pronouncements that sounded good on paper, but for one reason or another were difficult, if not impossible to pull off in "real" life, was a waste of everybody's time. Americans want very badly to be thin. They will resort to some of the wildest, most idiotic schemes imaginable if they're fast and easy. We like a lot of things fast and easy, don't we?

Just like any scientist that experiments on himself for the purpose of furthering science, I kept a journal of my personal experiences on the weight loss trail. The great thing about this is, as you will soon see, it didn't take superhuman abilities to get the body I have today. You will also see that no uphill climb is straight up. There are thoughts and ideas contained in the journal that are not directly related to weight loss, but do pertain to developing the life we all long for. This is assuming, of course, that you long for the much heralded, the much vaunted, and generally expected American Dream. The one where life is fun and easy, where we're all beautiful people, and you get all that you hope for.

One thing I've learned through all this is that being in charge of your own destiny, captaining your own ship, and feeling like you're doing a good job of steering, sure helps bring those allusive qualities of the good life a little closer. That's what THE FABULOUS SEX ORGAN DIET helps you do. It helps you to gain the distinct feeling that things are going to work out as you begin to take charge of your life. As you read the following pages, I hope you'll take heart in the fact that while there is no magic formula, THE FABULOUS SEX ORGAN DIET is about as close as it gets in this, or any other life, to a diet many people feel is a piece of cake!

DAY 1

I have decided to start keeping a journal of my experiences on what I believe is a totally new and improved weight loss program. These excellent thoughts shouldn't be kept from my progeny, especially in the event that the next 30 days prove to be the death of me. Developing this program has been totally radical, and if it doesn't work, I'm going to be totally pissed. Is it too much to ask to lose weight, shape up, and gain control of one's life in thirty days? It better not be.

My expectations as to just what I can expect from my life have varied somewhat with the passage of time. Even though I've been reasonably successful financially, and despite overcoming an untold number of obstacles to get this far in life, the feeling of being in control of my life has always been rather elusive. It seems like there's always something cropping up to derail me, whether early on or well into a project.

This program will hopefully be different. What I would like to accomplish initially is to gain control over my dietary habits within the thirty day period, and broaden that control as the ability to direct my course improves. In launching this brand new ship of life, I've decided to take a page from the world class high jumpers. I actually got the idea from all the New Year's resolutions I've made, and the more I thought about it, the more I realized that many of the world's most successful athletes do the same thing. The idea, as adapted, is to set a target date for the beginning of the program, and get a running start. I seem to have a great deal of momentum in January, and I think it's because I spend the whole month of December telling myself that come the New Year, I'm going to do thus and so, and start planning for it. Anyway, since I'm bound and determined to direct the course of my new ship instead of letting it drift along, circling around in a sea of despair until I run out of steam, I decided to get a running start. As such, while this is the first day of the actual diet and exercise program, I've been preparing for this for about three weeks.

The first question that comes to mind as I embark on a journey that's sure to change my life forever is: Why have I decided at this particular time to launch what many experts feel is a key turning point in my life? As far as I can see, many really smart people have been skirting around the idea of a sex organ diet, but nobody's nailed it like I think I have. Can I create something that changes my life and changes others by example? That often seems to be the nature of dramatic discoveries!

I have just turned 39. For my birthday, I asked for, and received, a beautiful new vasectomy to prevent the addition of another child to my already bulging family. I married a young woman because I've always felt that a man is only as young as the woman he feels. But in spite of all attempts to insure that my wife's uterus was fully covered in case of accidental entry, I have been unable to stem the onslaught of children. This has lead to an utter disappointment in the infallibility of modern birth control methods. The first baby was a failure of the pill. The second was diaphragm failure. Using that thing was like beating your head against a wall, it had to go. It was just one of those wacky ideas that came and went. Unfortunately it went before I came. Thirdly, not more than two weeks after the installation of an IUD, our next and hopefully last child was ill conceived. If I have another, after having whole sections of my body removed, for-get-it. I will not, under any circumstances, remove my trouser snake. That's too much to give, even for science. I just can't believe how incredibly fertile I am!

Getting back to why this diet has suddenly become so pressing an idea. I think it's the ten year cycle. I have strong evidence to suggest that major changes have transpired in my life every year ending in zero, since I was nine (1960), and my Mom got Leukemia and went away to the hospital. There also seems to be a five year subcycle dating back to 1967 when my Dad died, and a four year mini within the two.

I don't know if the major changes that seem to happen with such great regularity in my life are by chance or by design. But it's clear to me that virtually all of the big changes in my life have happened at extremely regular intervals, and this appears to be coming right on schedule. The drive I feel to get this idea in the hands of an eager public seems like the compulsion Kevin Cosner's character had in the movie, <u>Field of Dreams</u>. It got him motivated to build a ball field, and when it came over him, it just didn't quit. I feel a big change coming and it's almost ten years to the day since the last one. It's kind of funny really, now that I think of it.

Well, whatever the reason, I can honestly say that I'm sick and tired of not being awesome anymore, and would like to be again. The idea of fading into mediocrity, sends chills down to my sphincter. If Arnold Palmer is correct, in that the harder he practices, the luckier he gets, it's time for me to get in gear and start practicing harder, cause I might need a little luck to pull this off.

The things I want to get accomplished on this thirty day extravaganza are as follows: First, I want to lose weight. I really am done being chubby. I weighed in at 227 lbs yesterday and I would like to be thirty pounds lighter. There's a great deal of self image tied up in how much I've weighted over the years. When I felt my best mentally, when I was really on top of my career, my body was at it's best. When I was down and felt wounded psychologically, I chubbed out physically.

It's hard to answer the question, "which has to come first?", but if I'm trim and energetic, my feeling of well-being will certainly improve my quality of life, even if my career doesn't. When I'm trim and my clothes fit well, I really look sharp, and business seems to go better. Maybe the answer really does lie in the power of THE LIFEFORCE found in sex organs.

Sex organs are life giving by definition, and seem to produce energy and good health in all who eat them. I think it best at this point that I limit my focus to sex organs of the plant world. Since sex organs of the animal kingdom have not demonstrated, at least to my knowledge, an accrual of any salubrious benefits upon ingestion, like plants' organs have.

The simple method of determining what can or cannot be eaten is done by asking oneself if what they're about to eat is a sex organ. If one were to eat only sex organs and vegetables it would obviously preclude meat from the diet. This alone would produce tremendous weight loss if continued long enough. The simple reason for this is that there just aren't any fat vegetarians, and that is essentially what you'd be. But simply saying "I'm a vegetarian" has no panache, no savior faire, and I want this to be striking. It needs to feel nouveau, and maybe a little avant garde, and yet hit the nail on the head.

Along with the diet I've planned an exercise program to get the blood circulating, but not be so hard as to be discouraging early on. I need to whip this flaccid tissue of mine into better shape. A regular schedule of exercise, along with the aforementioned dietary regimen, will not necessarily be easy. But if I can kick this thing into gear, the next ten years might be very productive.

But whether it's easy or hard, I really need to get my act together because the termites of life are eating me alive. My energy level is low, and my initiative is marginal at best. My willingness to share the duties of running a household littered with kids, doesn't seem to be there. All I've been able to do is thank God that he delivered unto me a wife of unparalleled quality. If I would have been forced to make due without her, having three kids in twenty seven months would have been much harder than it was. She's been a real saint, complete with plenty of patience during my long decent from earlier heights of glory. She will, however, be rewarded beyond her wildest dreams if I can figure out a fast and easy way to bring about a healthy thinning of America. After all, if modern science can finally figure out a way to thin paint, we should be able to figure out how to thin Americans. This diet has to be fun, and yet safe, in order to be effective. One that works for the long haul, and yet won't be like climbing Mount Olympus!

Day 2

The second day of this change of life is now more than half over and it's clearly working. The real test however, is almost certainly yet to come. Can I avoid the urge to eat sweets late at night? That's the question now facing me.

I think one of the real keys to this diet is going to be visualizing the way things are supposed to go, and to use graphic visual images to destroy yearnings for food by picturing it in some grotesque manner. What effect would it have on the desire for sweet rolls if instead of sitting there for fifteen minutes fantasizing about all of their wonderful qualities, I sat there and imagined cockroaches crawling all over them or visualizing, in graphic detail their being puked on by some stinking, stumbling, stammering drunk. A drunk so completely disgusting that his stench alone would keep you from those rolls. I've got to believe that if I can visualize having to clean off the vomit to eat them, they're going to end up being just a little less appealing than before I started. I believe that the appeal of cravings can be systematically destroyed by using these visualizations!

The day was well begun. I was up at 6:45, dressed and ready to exercise. I walked several miles through dense jungle to get to the donut shop (just kidding), and it only took 35 minutes. Fortunately, there were no dangerous beasts to fight off, as there would be in Manhattan. It was great to get out in the early morning air for the second time in years, and have the intuitive sense that I was doing something very worthwhile.

The nice thing about this diet is that you can eat literally as much as you can hold, any time you want, before noon. Lest I forget, let me make mention of the juice of sex organs as well. There's nothing that'll charge you up like a big glass of fresh juice from a sex organ. It's full of THE LIFEFORCE! Let me also make mention of the life giving properties of water. Water is the essence of every animate thing on the planet. Life can not function without it and I get the feeling from my doctor that none of us drinks nearly enough. HE says that staying hydrated, as they say in the bizz, is critical to weight loss and properly functioning parts. This I must pursue!

It has occurred to me that originating THE FABULOUS SEX ORGAN DIET at precisely this time in my erstwhile career as a human being, when I've just had a vasectomy, could be just a little bit Freudian. Perhaps it's some kind of transference or compensation. Who knows? I only know that I love the idea of eating sex organs. It all sounds so virile, and what an opportunity for the palate! When I wrap my tongue around a sex organ I can almost feel the weight falling off!

DAY 3

Three days in a row. The evidence that I may be on a roll is mounting. I've gotten up every morning this week and exercised. Of course, all this amounts to right now is walking a mile or two, but by golly I'm doing something I've never done before, which is getting up extra early and exercising, and it really feels great.

The plan is to walk the first week, then start riding my ten-speed the second. The third week I may add something else or I may not, I haven't decided. The quantity is not as important as the continuance right now. Getting out early in the morning and breathing the fresh clean air instead of laying in bed and dreading the thought of getting up and going to work - what a change!

One thing I want to end is the practice of falling asleep in my reading chair right after dinner. I have been conking out for an hour or so each day and while it really feels good, it can be construed as a bad habit. It stops the process of getting things done, of being productive in the evening, because once I wake up, all I do is read or watch the tube, no sex or anything.

Now in and of itself, this isn't altogether bad, but it is anti-social and isolates me from Lori and the kids. Since I'm away from them so much as it is (running the business), it might be better for the family if they had a chance to interact with dear ol' dad.

Come to think of it, one thing I need to do more of, all over the place, is to be more considerate of others. Maybe it isn't as much consideration as it is thoughtfulness. I think everyone must sense that it's important to SHOW care and concern for those we care for and are concerned about. It seems so important to be a man of action and get things done, but if I don't take more time to show thoughtfulness now, while I can, I might lose an opportunity forever. You never know when someone you care about is going to cash in their chips.

A guy I've known for years and years, just got blindsided by a substantial truck. Now he's dead and gone, and he was a young guy. I'm sure all his many friends thought they'd have thirty or forty more years to tell him how much they liked him. But no more! That's why I'm convinced that it's best not to leave thoughtfulness for some future time that may never arrive.

And another thing, since I want this program to elevate not only my body, but my mind and soul, to the new plateau I foresee, do I need to add more layers to this program? What is the best way to become a man of action? A man who seizes the day, as Robin Williams might say, and constantly goes after that which is important to him. I believe that what I need desperately is to live with passion, energy, and excitement. The difference between charging forward, and grasping the nettle with verve, as you pluck it from the ground, and gingerly gripping it with fear and trembling, being painfully stung in the process, as the story goes, is the gusto with which you attack it. How important is it to live with gusto?

DAY 4

So far the whole process seems to be going according to plan. Getting up every morning seems to be getting a little easier. That's one of the great things about this whole plan.

If I become a morning person, I should become more efficient, almost by default. I have the ability to get things done, what I want is the will and the determination to go after what I really want.

There are some additional habits I would like to acquire, and one of them is regularly listening to motivational tapes by some of America's most inspirational and thought provoking speakers. I have found them of great value in the past, particularly Dennis Wheatley and Earl "the Pearl" Nightingale. They help to focus in on just what it is we want. Then they detail practical, proven methods for accomplishing those wants. Their effect however is not necessarily permanent, unless the listener is prepared to follow through. They can give us a jump start to help break the inertial bounds that encumber us, if we're beings at rest. But when it comes down to the short hairs, we are the ones that must do what it takes. Fortunately, once we become relentless, it's no problem!

I guess I think the tapes work best for me if I listen to them as many times during the day as possible, over and over, until their words permeate my thoughts. At that point, the input begins to achieve the desired output. I think it probably gets back to this: "We become what we think about," and once the tapes reorder our thinking, the auto-pilot makes that turn onto the new course. The nice thing about these guys is that they've got tons of useful suggestions that go far beyond the simple Rah -- Rah approach to motivation. They don't input mindless pep, but ways that help make permanent change possible.

DAY 5

Walking is getting easier, and if you ask me it's too easy. I've enlisted my neighbor to get up with me and work out. There is no question but that finding a partner helps perpetuate the exercise routine, particularly in the beginning, when the possibility of bagging it is the greatest. When there is a little bit of peer pressure to keep one moving forward, it makes a difference, it really does. Just as an example, I can think of a lot of stuff I'd never get to if it weren't for my wife. She's a real motivator, that woman!

My partner, Steve, is going to start riding a bike with me on Monday, which should produce increased sweat and energy expenditure. Since we both enjoy being big spenders, we're going to see how much energy we can spend.

Tomorrow night we have to attend a big kickoff dinner for the Airshow, and the meal almost certainly will not be all sex organs. So what I'm going to do is sneak home before the dinner and have a big bowl of vegetable soup. That way when we go to the dinner, I won't be hungry and consequently feel compelled to eat the flesh of animals. I'll report back on how this strategy works out.

DAY 6

We missed our workout this morning because of rain. While walking in the rain is romantic if you're Gene Kelly, if you're not, it's just wet. So we talked each other into baggin' it. We'll pick it up a notch Monday morning however (next week), when the reconditioned ten-speed (actually it's an eighteen speed, but thirteen or fourteen of those gears are wasted on me) hits the road.

Went to the Airshow Dinner and it was a buffet style dinner, so it was easy to decide what I was going to eat. I did, however, have that bowl of soup before going, and it worked perfectly. I wasn't hungry when it came time to eat, so I really didn't feel compelled to chow down.

So RULE # 33, PRE-EAT SOMETHING LIGHT ABOUT AN HOUR BEFORE THE MEAL IF YOU DON'T WANT TO CHOW DOWN AT THE MEAL ITSELF!

I did eat a big plate of sex organs in public, but nobody seemed to take umbrage. The Sex Organ Diet is a real shocker to talk about over dinner however. I just casually mentioned that I was on The Sex Organ Diet and I was immediately the center of attention at our table. People really aren't sure what I'm talking about, but they are sure that there must be some explanation, and they want to hear it. It definitely has a mystique about it. I still wonder about the timing of THE FABULOUS SEX ORGAN DIET, coming as a flash of sheer genius right after the vasectomy. It still feels Freudian, but it's working. Maybe it's more along the line of thought developed by Sigmund's brother, French.

One footnote to the dinner: I decided to have a piece of carrot cake after tasting a piece of my wife's. That was a big mistake, tasting my wife's I mean. I had absolutely no interest in having any (my resolve was quite high) until I had that taste in my mouth. It was soooo good that I decided, of my own free will, to embrace the experience with gusto, and live on the wild side.

Needless to say, the Carrot Cake, or the Cheese Cake that followed (which was also very good, but which I only ate part of) is not going to destroy either my resolve or my diet, because I am bound and determined! It will however, slow it down for an evening. But I guess dieting is like ten speeding, sometimes you have to downshift to get over those hills!

RULE #45, IT IS MUCH BETTER NOT TO TAKE THE FIRST TASTE, RATHER THAN HOPE TO EAT ONLY A LITTLE OF SOMETHING THAT TASTES GREAT AND IS AVAILABLE IN QUANTITY!

DAY 7

We didn't do any exercising this morning because Steve's an Airshow volunteer and had to be there at 7:00 A.M. But I did think of my first vegetable joke and I must record it for posterior. What do you get when you cross a penis and a potato? Answer - A Dictator! I'm probably not in any danger of being sucked dry as a Hollywood writer doing this kind of stuff, but a few more like that and my name will probably be etched in vegetables.

Later in the day, my lovely bride and I took a long walk in order to keep this fitness thing going. After the walk, we went to the Airshow and walked some more. I didn't like walking around with a protruding belly hanging over my belt. Not only is it not me, it's not the image I want to project. It's not the image that tells people who and what I really am as a person. The old saw about never getting a second chance to make a first impression is of course true, and when we care about what others think of us, which seems to be fairly natural, we should make every attempt be what we think we are, not what others think we are. That's why I'm really glad I'm going to be slim. It feels good to have my clothes fit well. I want it and I mean to have it!

I used RULE #45 to great effect at the Airshow. Just as we were getting hungry, after walking around for a while, Lori stumbled upon multiple bags of free chips at one of the courtesy tents, and brought back an armfull. After just having learned a valuable lesson the day before, I decided not to have "a few" and save myself for dinner. Not having the first certainly meant that I couldn't possibly have a second.

DAY 8

Today has been a fairly laid back episode. After going to Church and thanking God for sex organs, I came home and had breakfast. We then went over to a client's house to see the latest blooms in her flower garden and eat a late lunch. Boy that woman has quite a spread. She's got a real fertile pasture, and I suspect there's been quite a few that had it occur to them that it'd be a right nice little patch for grazing, and her flowers are nice too. Why she's so charming, I just wanted to pull her aside and talk to her about the pleasure to be had in eating sex organs, like I've been doing, and how great it could make her feel. She's the kind of woman that would really enjoy something like that. Unfortunately, I never really got the chance with so many people there. But no matter how you cut it, she certainly is a fabulous woman! It's really too bad she's over eighty.

As an overview of the first week, I feel it went fairly well in some areas, after all, I did write two rules. But there are, as one might expect for a program this early in it's life cycle, areas that need work. I want to be more energetic, more vital, and more alive. I want to be more attentive to my personal habits, and more productive over all. I wonder if it would be of any real value to keep a log, or a daily record, of all the things I accomplish each day, in order to measure my productivity? I guess I'm proud of the start I've made. I think the running start idea can take the credit. I'm proud that I squeezed getting up early into my busy schedule and that I did my walking come "clouds or shine." I'm very happy with the feeling I get, filling myself with THE LIFEFORCE found in sex organs. Can true success be far away? Not if I maintain the focus of a Laser beam!

DAY 9

Got up and rode the bike for a half an hour this morning and it felt tremendous! Boy, I'll tell ya, getting that morning air in my lungs, and smelling the fresh scents from the morning blooms as I rode was almost cosmic. Steve couldn't ride this morning so I didn't have someone pushing me forward, but it was cool, and tomorrow it'll be even better.

Riding seems more fun than walking. For one thing, you can coast and still move forward. Coasting while you're walking brings your net forward progress to a virtual halt. However, one thing about coasting that an old business associate, Bill Mueller, told me, is still very relevant today. He used to tell me is that you can only coast down hill, and that's exactly where you're going when you do coast. "Good point", as Jim Moshenko, a good friend of mine would say.

The only thing I have to lament about riding ten speeds is the nature of the seat. It seems to be built for very light castratos with other things on their mind, as one would expect. It's definitely a pain, but Steve said it'll make us hard asses, and what could be better than that? After riding for five minutes my little noogies were saying, "John, John, John, think it over buddy! We're still tender vittles from the ol' vasectomy! Think of us for a change would ya?" I have been able to think of little else for the past several weeks, and made a mental note to tell them both to go get screwed. I thought it would be best for all concerned.

DAY 10

I would've loved to have gone back to bed this morning but I kept my momentum moving forward, and got up. We went about six miles in half an hour on the bikes. It was quite refreshing and, once in the saddle, most of me was glad I got up. One thing I've noticed is that following through will always gain one the respect of one's peers. Provided, of course, they're not fundamentally opposed to what you're trying to do. Even then, it is still possible to earn their grudging admiration if you're deft at following through. If one could always follow through on one's efforts, one would become extremely powerful, because the world is in short supply of people who can absolutely be relied upon to follow through!

DAY 11

Getting up this morning, after last night's Piston's game was the hardest challenge yet. But once again I followed through and came out a winner. I sure hope all this effort is going to translate into lost weight, because I'm certainly not doing this for my health!

I've noticed a little bit of diet violation creeping into my daily affairs. It's difficult to know how rigid one should be with one's self. After making a personal decision to forgo coffee, I had two cups today and they both tasted great. In choosing immediate pleasure, over the longer term good I became short sighted. Perhaps one important aspect of temporarily forgoing a valued goal is the transcendence of the immediacy of the moment above all else.

The craven tendency to put short term pleasure ahead of reasoned judgment and long term gain is a childlike (or childish) quality. How does one throttle the pleasure sense so that at key moments, the impulse to abandon stated objectives can be easily subdued, without the traumatic loss normally associated with forgoing a pleasure.

Is the question then: How do we make self discipline easy and enjoyable? Is self discipline what we're really talking about here, or is it something else? Can one transmute the pleasure sense, for the sake of ultimate gain, without being self disciplined?

I feel, and this has been corroborated by other experts in the field, that the battle of the will versus the driving nature of the pleasure sense is determined by the nature of visualizations inputted at the moment of temptation. If I send a strong visualization of the wonderfulness of the pleasure first, it gets anchored and becomes difficult to remove because it keeps playing until we've either suppressed it or given in. I think it's better to have prerecorded messages already stored, ones that will be cued up and played automatically, at the instant the thought occurs to us to do something that isn't best. This way the pleasure sense can be anchored to an entirely different outcome.

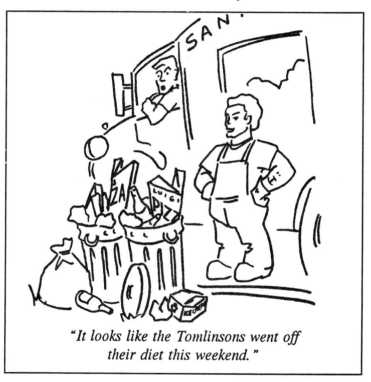

"It looks like the Tomlinsons went off their diet this weekend."

Setting a mechanism in place which will anchor what is pleasurable (in light of over all wants), rather than the fleeting urges spawned by the palette, makes the most sense. It's important to see to it that pleasure is derived, not from falling in the pothole, but from missing it. As man has so aptly shown us over the ages, pleasure can be milked from almost any act or series of acts. We decide! That's the beauty of using strong visualizations to pre-set the outcome of occurrences or actions (prompted by thoughts popping into our heads) that aren't in line with what we really want. We can deal with them before they end up pitting one half of us against the other half, in a conflict that is sure to create angst.

DAY 12

When I got out to ride this morning there was lightening and thunder all over the place. I decided to go anyway. I figured that it might pass, and if it didn't, I'd turn around at the first sign of serious drops and sprint back. It was quite a sprint!

I'm finding more and more, that eating no meat is reasonably simple. I don't crave it, and I certainly don't need it. I miss foods like hamburgers, pizza, and barbecued ribs. But in time those may not matter either - Yeah right! The key will be balance. Eating the various foods that we've come to enjoy, once we've reached our objective, is different than eating things that push our goals further into the future.

After I've crossed the river, having traversed the swift and swirling currents, I can kneel down at the water's edge and get a drink if I happen to be thirsty. No problem. But if I stop in the middle of the river, let go of the line, and put my hands down to take a drink, it becomes a somewhat more perilous an act on my part. Rather than doing the smart thing and waiting until I'm safely across, I could end up jeopardizing the entire crossing if I take my eyes off the distant shore and bend down to drink. It sets up the possibility, as one can easily see, of getting swept up by the current and washed away. Therefore, it makes sense to forego what ever prevents me from getting to the shore, where I really want to be, drink or no drink.

Since the diet, as it currently stands, allows me to eat anything that is a product of a sex organ, I've been having a peanut butter and jelly sandwich almost every night. I'm not sure this is a good idea. My doctor says that peanut butter is high in cholesterol, and yet it's from a sex organ. Must be the wrong sex. I'll research it further and report back later.

DAY 13

Didn't make ten speeding this morning because of those damned Pistons. It was a very late game, and staying up to watch them win was no trouble, and what a win it was. Down by seven with two minutes left, they scored the last nine points in a row, hitting the winning basket with seven tenths of a second left on the clock to clinch the title. What a game. It sure was a workout. I didn't have much left at the end.

The diet is getting easy. I've resigned myself to eating only sex organs, and so far I haven't felt tempted much. It really is becoming clear that a lot of temptation stems from fantasizing about the pleasure one would have if one were to indulge oneself in the fantasy of the moment. If the visualization is sterilized, so that it loses it's reproductive powers of attraction, the yearning will be rendered impotent.

DAY 14

I felt the urge to exercise today, but was able to suppress it. I rendered the desire impotent with sophisticated mind control techniques. This visualization stuff is really working.

DAY 15

This is getting scary. I rendered impotent my burning desire to do work around the house. No kidding! I got up this morning with a huge list of jobs and before you know it, all desire was gone. It simply vanished, and it was all I could do to find the strength to watch movies all day. It's like a miracle!

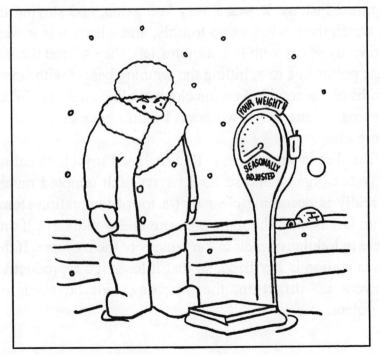

DAY 16

We hit the trail bright and early this morning and I feel the momentum building again. Steve has lost 15 lbs so far and is ecstatic. He's now so excited about eating sex organs that he can't control himself. He thinks about 'em all day. I must ask him just what his favorite sex organ is. I would guess that he has probably narrowed it down to one or two. I'll bet he's got a hot tip he'd like to share. I know his dear wife is excited about his being on this diet. Every time I see her she has this really big shit eatin' grin on her face. I'm sure it's because he's losing all the weight. But maybe it's because of all that vigor and vitality he's acquired!

I, on the other hand have only lost nine pounds, and while my clothes are definitely fitting better, I want to lose a lot more. I wonder if it would help to change sex organs. I've been eating a lot of beans, much to the disappointment of my friends and countrymen, and maybe they're too heavy. One thing I know for sure is that there are no fat vegetarians. So perhaps I'm being a little impetuous here. I feel great, I am losing weight, I've got much more energy in just a couple of weeks, and I am getting excited about making it happen instead letting it happen. Maybe I'll just keep working hard and be a little bit more patient with myself. It's not important that it happen overnight, it just has to happen.

DAY 17

I didn't make it up this morning, but it wasn't my fault. My dear, darling Lorinda got up at five to do some work for her graphic design business and didn't reset the alarm. So I decided to take a walk after work and enjoy some of that delicious sunshine I miss all day. It really feels great to get outside more. When I was a kid, you couldn't keep me in the house. I was either playing some sport or out playing in the woods. Maybe it's time I took the time to go out and play a little bit. Maybe I need to let the kid out a little more...

I'm starting to experience the flushing of my system. Taking a dump is a brand new story when you're recycling sex organs. The roughage seems to move the trapped sediment through the system. I'm seeing things I haven't seen in years. As a matter of fact, I read that by the time meat eaters are fifty, they have as much as five pounds of undigested red meat in their intestines. What a mess huh?

DAY 18

Again, no bicycling today, but it was because of a Board Meeting at the Art Institute. So I took another walk, only this time in another direction. It's like going exploring because everything seems to take on a different perspective when you're walking, as opposed to zipping by in a car. Going by the pond and hearing the frogs chirp and the birds sing, or is it the birds that chirp? Anyway, suffice it to say that you really don't notice how much of the world you miss while being safely locked away in the ol' auto, when contact with the world is sealed out. You think you know, but it's easy to forget I guess.

Still, I'm not happy about missing my morning ride two days in a row. It won't happen tomorrow, I'll see to that! Something good happened tonight. I was just sitting around watching the tube and I got inspired to do some exercises.

I did some sit-ups, leg lifts, side leg lifts, push-ups and jumping jacks. Then I got the idea to put on one of my favorite albums, Styks' "Paradise Theater", and started hoppin an' boppin around the house. It was great! Absolutely great! At first the kids looked at me like I was a little weird. But the music is so infectious that pretty soon they were hard at it as well. Then the Misses joined in and it was a dance. We laughed and sweat and got pumped.

I think that's going to happen a lot more often in the future than it did in the past! I think riding every morning does more than just make me sweat. It gets the deep breathing going and, as that rich oxygenated blood swirls around the brain, it creates a feeling of well being. The worries of the day are melted away before they get a chance to build up and my self confidence is improving, just knowing that I'm following through on a program that takes a little effort. I'm getting personally excited here!

DAY 19

Had a great ride today! We're starting to stretch it out and it feels better all the time. I see big weight loss ahead. If I can continue this pace, I'll be a stick by the end of the summer. What do I mean if? I'm doing it and that's all there is to it!

An interesting angle came to me today when thinking about why I haven't felt any desire for foods that aren't part of the diet. In trying to fathom why I've not been bothered by either the desire for the flesh of animals or the need for sweets, I realized in a sudden flash of illumination that it's all in the power of the sex organs I've been eating! It's THE LIFEFORCE at work!

You would think that I would have realized the power of this force after having three kids in twenty seven months, in spite of all attempts to impede the white hoard, but no. I didn't realize the true cosmic power of sex organs until I started gorging myself on them (fruits) to the exclusion of all else, till noon.

I think the secret lies in the tremendous satisfaction offered by the sex organ itself. Once you take in this LIFEFORCE every morning, you start to sense that your needs are being fulfilled, maybe for the first time, while your body just keeps getting skinnier.

A fruit, according to my research, is the fertilized ovary of a plant, grown from a flower. The seed or seeds are self-contained within the unit. Due to the embryonic nature of fruit, it's a unit for reproducing a life form and as with humans, the area between the outer cover and the core is mostly water. A ripe tomato, as an example, can be as much as 97% water. The life giving nutrients contained in that area of the fruit spawn incredible growth, and in humans, it produces tremendous vigor! Fruits, as a category, include many more items than you would think. Tomatoes, of course, are fruits, but so are peas, cucumbers, beans, squashes, corn, nuts and many things that are referred to as vegetables. Vegetables, on the other hand are defined as ANY eatable part of a plant. This would include, roots, stems, stalks, leaves, flowers, buds and also fruits, which are themselves a subset of vegetables.

I wanted to make mention of this because it isn't widely known by the average non-scientist. I should add at this point, however, that horticulturists (people who study the science and art of growing fruits, vegetables, flowers, and ornamental plants) consider only the fertilized ovary of a perennial as a fruit. A perennial is a plant that continues to grow year after year, as opposed to plants that must be replanted each year their fruit is desired. Wasn't it Dorothy Parker who once said," You can lead a whore to culture but you can't make her think!" The whole thing was that they didn't need to be concerned with thinking, but you can bet they were eating sex organs!

The point I was going to make before I got sidetracked was that fruits are filled with naturally occurring sugars in great quantities. So as a direct result of getting all this sugar in the blood, your body feels like it's got all it needs, and it's very unlikely to crave more. As a consequence, the natural cravings one might experience for quick sources of sugar, like cakes, pies, donuts, cookies, pop and candy seem to vanish.

Here's a test that I can challenge anyone with. Have them sit down and eat a half a watermelon, or any kind of melon for that matter, and watch their desire for confections melt like butter over hot croissants. The beautiful part of eating all this natural sugar is that you feel more energy than if you drank a big cup of coffee, and more clarity of mind than if you've been drinking scotch all day!

DAY 20

This bicycling thing is starting to get in a groove. The psychological benefits of getting up early and doing something seriously constructive before work are extensive. I have a clear feeling that I'm starting to gain control of my life. Taking extra steps to accomplish something seems to carry through to everything else done the rest of the day. I'm hoping that this momentum will carry through to other areas of my life, and enable me to really get my act together. With my energy level continuing to increase, my momentum and need are going to produce a force to be reckoned with. I just hope nothing derails what appears to be a marvelous effort.

DAY 21

I think I'm on to something! (I wonder if I'm starting to sound repetitious?) Once working out becomes a habit, it's like a boulder rolling downhill. The forces of nature, in this case gravity, keep it rolling. By the way, do you know the opposite of gravity? It's comedy. Think about it. Anyway, the air is freshest in the morning because the pollutants have settled. I think it has to do with the fact that the convection currents coming off the ground to produce rising air, subside after dark, when the surface is no longer being heated by the sun's ultra violet rays. So being heavier than air, the particles fall to the ground, or are washed to the ground in the case of rain. Ever wonder why your car is so dirty after it rains, even though your car just got a shower? It's because the raindrops picked up the dirt on the way down.

Thunderstorms have an even more pronounced effect on the air than ordinary rain storms. It's because of their electrical nature. Did you know that lightening bolts weigh in at forty thousand volts per inch, and as such, contain hundreds of millions of volts per bolt. This huge electrical generator charges all the little particles and particulates that are literally too small to fall, so they stick together like magnets and plunge to the earth, making the air incredibly fresh.

The first thing in the morning, the morning blooms produce a fragrance area, very similar to what happens in a room after a woman puts on perfume. It eventually gets dispersed when the cars start whizzing by. But until then, the world smells like a wonderful place. I wonder how many people actually take the time to enjoy the morning before getting ready for work. I'm probably late in this discovery, yet I can't help but think that with the fast pace of late twentieth century life, everybody's life has probably been zooming by like mine has, and the subtleties of life are lost in the shuffle. It's too bad. Maybe if more people took more time to appreciate the simple beauties, this world would be... Naaawww!

My eyes, however, are opening to a life I haven't had much chance to experience up til now. I wonder what other important things I'm missing? Am I starting to gain a new perspective on life as the forties loom just over the ridge, or is this the effect of constantly filling myself with THE LIFEFORCE from all those wonderful sex organs I've been eating? Whatever the reason, the LIFEFORCE found in fresh fruits and vegetables apparently cannot be minimized as a force for rejuvenation. I wonder if going on this diet is going to turn me into a philosophy student? Haven't you always been, even from the beginning, weedhopper?

This renewed philosophical interest has definitely had an effect on my work. I now love work. In fact I love it so much that I could sit and watch it all day, it's fascinating! But I've probably been watching it too much. I better slow down some. Maybe I should ease into the slow lane a little bit and catch some of the beauty that's been rushing past.

DAY 22

Sex organs have been on my mind a lot lately and I'm not talking about the one's you get at the produce department. I wonder if it's because it's spring, or if it's that damned LIFEFORCE again, welling up inside me, signaling that it's time to mate. Anyway, I was walking around campus today and was reminded of a quote by one of my favorite wits, Dorothy Parker (1893-1967). She said, during a commencement address, something to the effect that after walking around campus all day, and seeing all the beautiful co-eds, that if they were laid end to end, it wouldn't surprise her one bit. I kind of get the same feeling.

Over the years, a great deal of research has been put into having sex and sexual arousal, but I still don't have the full answer. I've often tried to put my finger on it, but they won't let me. I don't know why partially clothed mammary glands, with a feel that is somewhere between loose belly fat and a filled water balloon, can illicit such a strong internal response. Or why great female shapes produce such feelings of desire to reach out and touch someone.

But it is powerful enough that virtually everything advertised uses sex to get people to buy, and you know what? It works like crazy. My doctor told me that he had to hook up a twenty four hour heart monitor to a patient complaining of chest pains. The patient had to write down everything he did so that they could correlate what he was doing with his heart rate. The interesting thing was, according to the doctor, the guy's heart raced faster during the anticipation phase, when he was just thinking about what he was going to be doing with his wife, then when he actually had the sex.

Come to think of it, I'm not sure whether that's a comment on the effects of visual stimulation or the guy's sex life. I'd better research this further. "Honey, can you come here for a minute...?"

There must be a strong chemical released into the bloodstream upon receiving the visual stimuli, that drives the desire mechanism. The interesting thing is that what constitutes a visual stimulus for one person, can be completely different for another. This is not only true now but has been true throughout recorded history. Going all the way back to the ancient Greeks, as an example, we find that Plato used to complain bitterly about how goofy and irresponsible his best young philosophy students became around a winsome maid. It apparently really irked him, because he is quoted in the ancient texts as saying, "Love is a grave mental disease." We can draw two conclusions from this. First, this sexual arousal stuff has been around for as long as people have been making people. Two, is that it sounds like Plato hung around those Greek Baths just a little bit too much. Actually, I think Freud's courageous stand on sexuality was closer to the mark than many gave him credit for. Eating sex organs is sounding more and more natural all the time.

DAY 23

We tried to really drive ourselves on the bike today. There was a lot of huffing and puffing going up those somewhat modest hills, but after finishing we felt great. Scientists tell me that it's because the brain produces a group of strong narcotic substances called endorphins. During physical exertion they're responsible for the great feeling that settles over you when you sit down to rest afterward; and I understand that they're just as addictive as the ones available on the street a couple of blocks over. Can the ones available on the street a couple of blocks over. Can you believe it, just when I'm starting to exercise regularly and have fun at it, I find out that I might be getting addicted to it. Jeese, maybe I'd better quit this exercise stuff right now, and save myself while I still can!

Riding the bike is an aerobic exercise, which means breathing is important. Air, like water, is one of the few things we can't seem to do without and survive here on the planet (the others being, I believe, food and charge cards). How did people live before the discovery of plastic? It must have been a minimal existence. It's hard to imagine what it must have been like to actually have to earn money before spending it.

I think the first greatest discovery of the twentieth century was made by Einstein, during his research on time. Once he proved that time IS money, the development of the Mall seemed inevitable for those with a little time on their hands and no place to spend it. The second greatest discovery was that with the advent of plastic, we learned how to take our next two months at work, and compress it into an afternoon at said Mall. Scientists in Detroit made a quantum leap in time theory some time ago, when they developed a method whereby years and years of one's future existence could be compressed into an afternoon with a car dealer.

So the lesson here must be that if we take Einstein's thinking on time, and apply it to our own lives, we know that: A) We're leaving a lot of money on the table, which we could spend on ourselves if we didn't piss away our time; B) finding time to exercise is like finding money, because when you're done you'll be spent. But when you throw in the fact that as a reward for your goodness, your brain will produce powerful narcotics to make you feel wonderful, and that life is worth living (a useful illusion), you have to agree that exercising is better than not.

Just as a post thought to the aforementioned, I've often felt that for people who are suicidal or emotionally troubled, working out a couple hours a day would probably get rid of the mess in short order. One can actually retain anger and emotional trouble like one retains water, the only difference is the retentive chemical used. Fortunately, these pesky chemicals can be literally destroyed with vigorous exercise. At some point the body will stop making them and then the old feelings will be replaced with new feelings. For those people who find that life isn't worth living, they would be hard pressed to continue to feel that way after basking in the rich glow of an Endorphin Brain Bath every day for a few months.

Look at it this way, if you can rinse away what's eating you at the same time you're burning up what you're eating, you end up eating what's eating you before you get eaten yourself. Thereby avoiding the necessity of having to eat the dog that this dog eat dog world has placed in front of you for sustenance. You can finally live happily in the knowledge that you're eating to live, not living to eat, and this will help to avoid being eaten by the termites of life. So Exercise!

DAY 24

My partner continues to lose weight faster than I do, but

then he has more to give. It is great to see this whole thing working so well, it's always exciting to be a part of a success. He really is chomping down the sex organs, and he credits them with the great strides he's making!

Went over to get him this morning to go riding and his wife got up out of bed to let me in. Boy, oh boy, is she a number in a peach satin thing-a-ma-jig just covering her tender loins. I, after running out of sex organs the day before, asked her if it was all right if I ate hers. She said, "Sure, they're in the fridge."

It's probably a good place to keep them, because if the LIFEFORCE in those sex organs wasn't kept cooled down, and as a result started to heat up, maybe even started to get hot, those guys would probably just blow off breakfast altogether, and I'd never be able to get him up to go riding. Actually, if the truth be known, I think it would be better for all concerned if his lovely wife was the one to get him up every morning. That way he's raring to go when I get there. Beyond that, the moral of the story is that it's probably a good thing to keep your sex organs chilled out until you're ready to eat them. That way they retain the maximum LIFEFORCE!

Frankly, I think Steve learned to do this years ago. He said he was constantly finding himself losing all interest in breakfast, once he discovered that his favorite sex organs were left out in the open air. After all, when your sex organs start heating up, why bother to eat? So he and his lovely bride just stayed in bed day after day, until finally he realized that if he didn't keep his sex organs chilled out, he would never get anything to eat in the morning, and he wouldn't have all the energy he needed to get through the day.

Steve is kind of an interesting guy. I can't believe all the kids he has. He said to me one time, "John, do you know what you call people who use the rhythm method?" "No what?" "Parents!" He said. Can you believe it? I had to tell him point blank that he better stop that rhythm method or I was going to have to take him off the diet. I didn't want to be responsible for what might happen to his wife if he kept filling himself with the LIFEFORCE on top of everything else he's full of. She's already a lean, mean, birthing machine and they're completely out of bedrooms (they live in a mansion no less)! He finally said okay, but I don't know... When you start thinking with your sex organs instead of about them, anyth' g can happen!

DAY 25

I haven't had any cravings for sweets in some time, and I'm sure it's due to the fruit. I think the ease of being able to give coffee a rest was also helped by eating fruit, not only because of the natural energy replacement, but because in using sugar for my coffee I developed a sugar habit as well as a coffee habit. In trying to quit previously, I found that my desire for anything sweet just mushroomed. But this time it didn't happen. The effect of quitting coffee is noticeable to me. I find that when I awake in the morning I don't lie there in a haze for a while, feeling like I need a little more rest before rising. I get up feeling rested. I also have much more energy after dinner than I used to, because I don't have to work through what I've come to call, "Coffee Burn." This is when all the caffeine has been metabolized (used up), and the body is left with a spent feeling that takes the form of suddenly being super tired. This is completely gone and it feels so good to have enough energy to be springy instead of just plain sprung.

Anyway, I'm certainly not saying that I'm never going to have another cup of coffee, although I may not. What I am saying is that I have to admit I feel better when I don't drink it for a while. I may, at some point, revert to some form of dramatically reduced consumption, because it isn't essential to be Spartan to be healthy, but health sure feels good.

DAY 26

Heard a guy on a talk show today discussing the importance of properly combining the foods we eat for maximum energy efficiency. Apparently it takes so much energy to digest food, that if we can help the process to become more efficient, the un-utilized energy remaining after the process is complete, becomes available for everything else we want to do. He maintains that this will help us to feel energized! His basic premise is that since the tissue found in meat and fish are broken down with a very strong acid, and starches are broken down with enzymes that are alkaline (the opposite of an acid). When these two types of food are eaten together, the acid and the alkali tend to neutralize each other and it takes much, much longer for the work to get done.

With the stomach wasting a great deal of the body's energy store in the tug and pull of mixing the chemical equivalents of vinegar and baking soda together, we get much more tired after eating than need be. As such, the talk show guy recommends not eating the two groups together. This way digestion will take much less time and you don't get the after meal sag. Proteins contained in vegetables can be digested by either acid or alkali, so it doesn't matter with which group they're eaten. In fact, he heartily encourages their consumption in quantity. Starches, as we know, are in such things as breads, rolls, rice, tubers (tubers are starchy roots like potatoes), noodles and pasta.

He had some very interesting things to say about milk as well (he didn't mention cookies), and dairy products in general, that I found quite revealing. I think I'm going to do some extensive exploration on these ideas because the energy gain motif is a common thread with my sex organ diet. But it's all going to have to wait for tomorrow because I'm beat and need to log some sag time before riding in the morning.

DAY 27

Well it won't be long now (said the monkey after he caught his tail in the meat grinder), til my thirty day test will be finished. Barring the unforeseen, which is always a factor, I would say that THE FABULOUS SEX ORGAN DIET is a tremendous success! Not only did I lose weight (about 18 lbs so far), but I feel tremendous. I can state categorically that I feel better than I've felt in years!

The question is: Can I, or rather will I, stay on this program after the thirty days are over, or will I go back to what I was before? Boy, that doesn't sound like much of a choice does it? Going back to what I was thirty days ago makes no sense at all. Further, it really has no appeal. I like what I am now more, and what I'm doing for myself now is more than I've done in years. I mean after all, give up the joys of the morning? Come on, be Syrian...

There is so much power in the feeling that I'm taking control of my life and doing something positive about my health, my attitudes and my future. The thought of going backwards doesn't appeal to me whatsoever. Just think, I owe all this to all the sex organs I've been eating raw. The LIFEFORCE is with me.

I think the most important aspect of this approach to becoming a better specimen is that it's a painless, and relatively simple approach to weight loss. I didn't have to ever go hungry. I didn't have to eat really boring foods or eat one of several foods repetitively over an extended period (so that the whole thing became a tremendous ordeal that I began to loath) When you don't have to be miserable to get healthy, how can one not choose health?

Which gets back to what the experts say, and that is that truly successful weight loss programs enable you to modify your behavior so that the old habits fade while the new ones transcend, leaving one a much different, and generally better feeling person than before -- not just temporarily relieved, but better. In that regard, the nice thing about THE FABULOUS SEX ORGAN DIET is that it's like an old friend. You can go at your own pace. The more you employ the ancient dietary principles, the better things get for you. If you have to move away for a while, they'll be there waiting when you get back. Just as obviously though, while the friendship doesn't suffer the test of time if you do move away, you're body might. But fortunately it isn't permanent, as these most natural of all principles will work every time they're used, so don't leave them unemployed!

The good feelings they produce will become increasingly important in living my life, I'm sure of it. If I drift, it won't be far, because I want to remain in life's flow and feel the

LIFEFORCE coursing through my veins, not stagnating in some dietetic backwater, losing what little time I have left here on the planet. The key is whether I want to be with the force or against it. As Luke Skywalker found out, you just can't turn your back on the force!

Can you imagine how wonderful life would be if all of a sudden Americans everywhere decided that gorging themselves on sex organs made complete sense, and devotion to it became a national pass time. I can just hear it now. Americans everywhere going over to the neighbor's every morning to get some sex organs because they've run out. I'm sure the neighbors would welcome them with open arms saying, "Sure, come on in, they're in the fridge, help yourself!"

DAY 28

The fourth of July isn't too far away at this point, and we're planning the seventh annual Rambo Bivouac at our place on Beaver Island. Every year's been very different, but they've always been fun. I remember when some jerk, who shall forever remain nameless, started a big bond fire with gasoline. What a spectacle! The flames were so high and the wind was blowing so hard, that once they reached a certain height, they bent a full 90 degrees. It turned out to be an "L" shaped fire, which wouldn't have been so bad if the "L" hadn't been pointed at the neighbor's place. I told them it was okay and not to worry, but you know how neighbors are, it's always something...

Anyway, I thought Beaver Island would be a wonderful place to launch THE FABULOUS SEX ORGAN DIET. If I can get a whole camp full of people eating sex organs simultaneously, Katie bar the door! There'll be nothing left of them. It'll be wild, unleashing that LIFEFORCE in combination with the fresh air. They'll return to the known world as mere shadows of their former selves, spent!

What kind of exercise should we do up there? It should be something interactive that everybody really enjoys, and they're good at. It should be something they would like to do all the time if they could. The problem is that bullshitting doesn't burn that many calories and can take forever to finish.

Maybe this year we'll call it "Intense In Tents" and let the Bivouac-er-offers figure out the best way to burn calories. I know I'm going to lay on the sand and look at the stars. By the way, I heard that in Hollywood it's just the opposite. Speaking of which, I was telling a friend a simple joke. I asked him, "Do you know the difference between life in America and life in Russia?" "No" he replied. "Well, in America it's dog eat dog, and in Russia it's just the opposite!" And he says, "I don't get it, eat dog eat?" Boy, these computer guys!

DAY 29

I'm nearing the finish line and it's getting exciting! Biking is pretty easy now (relative to when I started), and if it wasn't for the fact that we've got to go to work, we would've added some distance to our jaunt. The key in aerobic exercise is getting the air intake and the heart rate up at least 40% for at least twenty minutes, so the body undergoes a systemic change from its base state.

One cannot underestimate the importance of air in the lungs, the question is "How much is enough?" We use only a very small portion of our total capacity. Since that's the case, what happens to the capacity we don't use? It just sits there holding old stale air until called upon to expel it and take in more. When you're in shape, the body gets much more oxygen into the blood because more of the lung space is naturally utilized. This increases the feeling of well being, the amount of fat burned, and the energy level we have to work with.

Where does this oxygen go? It is transported by red blood cells to every living cell in the body. To be exact, there's almost a 100 trillion of them. These cells then put that oxygen in their little furnace, called the mitocondria, and when it's mixed with sugar and fat, it facilitates the "burn" to produce energy for the body. As you know, things don't burn too well without oxygen. Just like when we inject oxygen into a campfire to get it to burn hotter and brighter by blowing into it, getting more oxygen into the blood by breathing deeper and more often (as with aerobic exercise), makes those fires in each cell furnace burn better and much cleaner, and, for the purpose of weight loss, much longer!

Now, it doesn't take a rocket scientist to see that if each cell in your body is burning up more stored energy (read fat), and at a faster rate, the mass of the body has to diminish, until you eat yourself completely!

In a nutshell, aerobic exercise seems to have several positive effects, not the least of which is to get the brain to produce those endorphins that I've come to know and love. Another great benefit is that physical exercise is a formidable suppressant of the appetite. This means that after exercising for a while, not only do we take in less than we used to, but we burn up a bigger percentage of what we eat. So losing weight picks up speed. That's why, from the beginning of recorded history forward, mankind has so praised the salubrious effects of attending regular aerobics classes.

DAY THIRTY!!!

I made it and I'm personally excited! Have you ever heard of the old expression, 'I went on the thirty day diet and lost six days.' Well, I went for the first thirty days of a much longer dietary regimen, lost 19 lbs and found a better way to live. Filling my body with the LIFEFORCE, and exercising in order to energize my existence has worked. The fact is, in some ways there was absolutely nothing new in what I did. Thousands of people lose thousands of pounds in thousands of different ways. In the words of King Soloman, "There is nothing new under the sun." So, I'm not going to claim that I've gone where no man has gone before. I'm sure the healthy of this world, who used to make me sick with all their health, would say I should've been doing this long ago!

If anything, I've added a unique perspective to the science of weight lose with the startling discovery that eating sex organs every day is cosmic, and puts one in touch with the LIFEFORCE. Now granted, in some of the more severe cases of LIFEFORCE DEPLETION it's going to be calling long distance at first, (until it gets closer to home) and for smokers it's probably going to call collect. But it's going to be there for you. The fact that this program was so easy that even I could do it should tell you that even you can do it.

I can't say that I never cheated, but inevitably cheating became irrelevant, as I realized that the ease and enjoyment of doing the right thing produced such a satisfying feeling. After a while I lost interest in doing that which made no sense. Even though I placed no absolute restrictions on myself, and was free to go where my desires led me, I couldn't get away from the satisfying feeling sex organs gave me.

In wrapping up this journal, which I really enjoyed writing over the last month, I want to leave myself, and any future practitioners of THE FABULOUS SEX ORGAN DIET, with some thoughts to chew on when a sex organ is unavailable.

The first is on experts, especially health experts. I've always been taken with a news article from years ago out of the L.A. Times. It was about a general strike by all the doctors in Los Angeles County for something or other. The interesting thing about the story was not what they wanted, but what happened after they walked out. For the next five or six days, at the hospitals, during the time that the doctors were out on strike, the death rate of patients in hospitals in the county dropped, some would say that the change was substantial, in relative terms. Then, when the strike was finally settled and the doctors went back to work (because their patients needed them so badly), the death rate climbed back to the general average previously in effect.

The point of this true story is that we can do a great deal to heal ourselves when it's important to do so. Doctors are essential to modern health care, and have made life safer for us all. But in many cases, they are simply trying to fix that which is a direct result of what we've done to ourselves. The body contains all it needs to know in order to maintain a healthy, well balanced existence, if we'll just let it live.

Deadly germs surround us every day, yet they have no

effect on us. Why is it that one person catches something, but the other doesn't? Perhaps the answer can be found in the word disease. When you break it down, this word has two parts. The first is *dis-* and the second is *ease*. *Dis,* as defined in Webster's New Collegiate Dictionary means; "to deprive of." *Ease,* on the other hand is defined as; "the state of being comfortable." So in essence, what we get when we get *disease* is that we've deprived ourselves of the natural comfort our body gets from its own good health.

The important point here is that we want to retain ease and comfort! In case you've lost it, all that it takes to regain it is to begin to do the right thing, and keep it up. Eating right and staying thin are not as hard to do as they might, at first glance, appear. In fact, just the opposite is the case, because if we will forsake disease, our brains, which see to the care and feeding of almost 100 trillion cells body wide, can certainly figure out how much you're supposed to weigh -- just let it!

The sex organs that man and woman have craved since the dawn of recorded time have been craved for a very good reason. It's the pleasure and the energy available from eating them which has always made them desirable! It is very difficult for any living soul to pass on to their progeny all that they have learned during their years on the planet. Therefore, we can safely assume that the answers to mankind's innermost desire, how to stay lean and healthy, have been both found and lost a thousand times over the centuries. Fortunately, by the grace of the Almighty, I, John Van Reginald Tomlinson III have found them again. BEAVER ISLAND, HERE I COME...

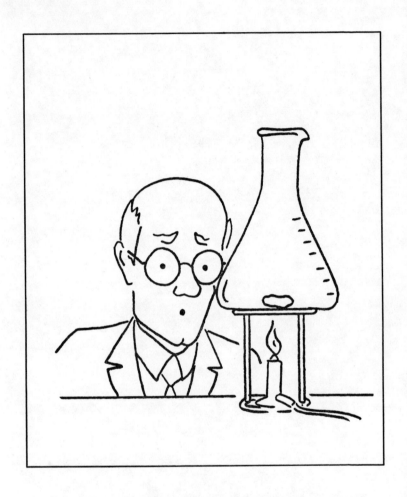

"What it all boils down to."

Chapter 8 -
THE END OF THE BEGINNING

The literature available today is mostly about having sex and very little about having children. Life, on the other hand, is the other way around. The same can easily be said for a number of other things we long to do but have very little time for, and as a consequence, end up reading about in hopes that someday the time will come to get down to it. However, in the mean time, reading about going on a diet can be a lot like reading about having sex. No matter how masterful the writer, it's never going to be the same reading about somebody else's orgasm.

Yet reading can be not only satisfying, but quite rewarding. The problem you face as a reader, is getting off the drawing board and putting your plan into effect. Fortunately, this is not a hard problem. All you need to do to begin is to pick a date. Use the beginning of the next month if it's no more than three weeks away or some other easily targetable date, and go for it! None of the things discussed, particularly those associated with the running start, require any will power or extra effort to get started!

The reason is that the running start takes place in your mind! All you need to do is pick the date and start purposefully and deliberately getting yourself excited about doing it. Think about it every day. In fact you should think about it constantly. Once the excitement you're pumping in, starts coming out, you'll find that the urge will come upon you to start the planning. When it does, run with it.

Remember, this plan need not be rocket science. You simply need to think through when, where, and how you're going to achieve an aerobic state for at least twenty minutes every day. You should start thinking about eating fruits every morning and think about properly combining your meals. But above and beyond all else, you must visualize relentlessly about becoming relentless in this pursuit. If there is one key, it is using your imagination to preprogram your actions and get yourself personally excited about the mission before the launch date!

Have you ever seen the movie "The Music Man?" Remember how during the whole movie he kept telling the kids that the instruments they were to play in the grand parade were coming and they shouldn't worry that they couldn't as of yet play them. What did he have them do to compensate for this drawback? Well, as you may remember, he had them continually going over their parts in their heads with such frequency and regularity that, coupled with how pumped he got them about the new uniforms and the beauty of the whole affair, when the time came to perform, they were brilliant!

Now I'm not going to suggest that what he did with those kids and their instruments was anything more than a good story told by some very talented people. But the point is absolutely unmistakable. He got the whole town so worked up about parade day (D-DAY) in their minds, that when it finally came to pass, they were ready, and you will be too! Just continuously input visualizations of every aspect of this new approach and let your mind do the rest.

Don't worry about if it's working or not. Think of this process the same way you think of planting flower seeds. You don't need to dig up the seeds every day to determine if they're sprouting and growing. You simply put them in, see to their care and feeding and pretty soon they'll start coming up. If you only put in one seed, it may or may not come up, because anything can happen to one seed. But if you plant a bunch of them, and keep planting them in different spots every day, in a few weeks you're going to have a ton of flowers! So remember, your first job is to plant as many seeds as you can possibly get in your acreage and keep planting them every day until you have a huge crop!

Think of getting started in this way and you'll find it incredibly easy to build momentum. If enough of the flowers come up early, you may feel the urge to push the starting date ahead. This is completely up to you. I would, however, urge you to consider the period of time between the commencement of your running start and D-DAY as a transition time. Continue to think in terms of gaining momentum for your D-DAY push. This way, you're sure to hit the ground running with such tremendous speed and force, that you'll blow by the barricades and be fifty yards down field before the opposition knows you've got the ball!

The beauty of this approach is that it takes no immediate work or extra effort on your part whatsoever. It takes no willpower, and you don't have to force yourself to do anything. You plant enough seeds and I guarantee you you'll have plenty of flowers come D-DAY!

I want to digress for a moment and re-examine the "old way" of losing weight. Sitting down to plan a new dietary regimen because you've suddenly gotten the urge to get healthy is difficult to do, and even harder to sustain. In fact, even though we're practically bombarded with things to read containing the salient benefits of a healthy diet, how many of us actually even read that stuff and get right on it? In all probability, unless you've had the proverbial "brush with death" which can be tremendously motivating (one that your current dietary regimen in all probability precipitated), eating right is usually quite a bit more conceptual than experiential.

The plain and simple truth is that getting motivated to endure the riggers of losing weight the old fashioned way (which has generally boiled down to eating various boring foods for ever, and even then getting precious little of it, while working your butt off at the gym until you almost feel like dying), is a bitch! Anyone who tells you it isn't, hasn't had to do it. The "come on you can do it" people are often found in the ranks of the perpetually skinny. They're the people who've always been on the seafood diet and it hasn't affected them - yet. You remember the seafood diet don't you? When you see food, you eat it!

For these reasons, I personally had to make a radical departure from the staid "Now eat your spinach" approach to dieting in order to be successful. Anybody in the world can stand up and say with great confidence that if you eat almost nothing and work your ass off at the gym for an extended period of time, you'll lose weight. Big deal! Losing weight after all, isn't rocket science. Everybody knows how. It's actually doing it, and even more importantly, continuing it until you've done what you set out to do, that holds all the glory!

Therefore, this book has never been about trying it for a couple of days and then tossing it on the stack with all your other diet books. It's about succeeding at something you truly want, but for one reason or another (and believe me the reason isn't even important anymore!) You've been thwarted in your drive to the goal line. Boiling failure down to a sports metaphor, we can see that we all fail for one of two reasons. Either we don't have much offense, or the defense is just too

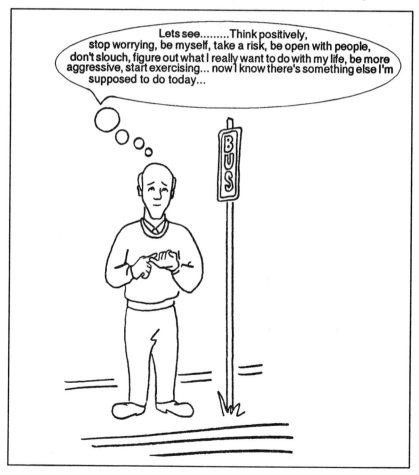

tough for our current offense. What we in effect do, with THE FABULOUS SEX ORGAN DIET, is to put in a completely new offense and show you how you can blow the defense off the field! Believe me, with this new game plan, as you learn to execute, you're going to score one hell of a lot of points and win the game by a wide margin!

There is one more play I want to put in to the complete game plan, but it's a secret play! This play is the key to having tremendous fourth quarter motivation when the defense is flat on it's back. It will give you that extra push that enables you to make sure that the other team (which I've decided to name Beaten Leftovers In My Past, or TEAM - B.L.I.M.P.), never gets back into the game. This secret play that will enable you to blow the BLIMPS into the bleachers and charge off the field like a champion! This one last play will give you the power to keep right on going as far as you want to go, in this or any other life!

The secret to motivation, as we long ago discussed, is to link the goal that you want to accomplish with a powerful emotion. The key is to find an emotion that is not only so powerful it will breathe tremendous invigoration into your goal, but it must be one that you're going to feel just as strongly three months from now as you do today. If the propellant is completely sprayed out of an aerosol can, even if the can is still half full, nothing else is going to squirt out. Similarly, if the emotion you choose to empower your goals (disgust motivation, which we talked about earlier, is a classic example of this very point) fades or dissipates, it loses it's ability to propel you toward your goal just when you're ready to score!

For that reason, I want to take a minute to talk to you about the sustaining power of your sex drives. Sexual association is the most consistently powerful motivating force in all of humanity, as Madison Avenue has so profitably found! The pull of sex and lust is almost without parallel in history. Furthermore, it is a force that will not desert you several months from now, when you're ready to blast the BLIMPS off the field forever. Even if down the road you "feel" differently about everything else in your life, your sex drives are going to be there for you. In fact, as you get healthy and fit, they're likely to increase substantially before your very eyes! If it can launch a thousand ships, it certainly should help you to cast off a few pounds!

Sex has always been a prime motivating force for me. Many of my earliest memories center around it. In fact, if you can believe this, I was even born in bed with a woman. The experience was so moving for the both of us, that for years after she was my love-slave and took care of my every want. The event had such an impact on me, that from that point in my life until this very moment, I've had an intense desire to return to the womb. Anybody's.

Unfortunately, it's not enough to have a tremendous sexual desire, because the whole secret isn't just having it, it's channeling it! Take the Colorado River, or even the Niagara. No power was ever gotten from either of those mighty rivers until the force within them was harnessed. To keep the propellant force behind your project, you've got to tie your goal to a force that you're sure is going to be there months or even years from now. You want a force that will continue to flow out of you indefinitely, like a mighty river, not a drainage ditch that will dry up when the rain stops. Anger would be a classic example of a drainage ditch emotion. If you tie yourself to the fleeting emotions that arouse strong feelings for a while, but fade and dissipate as the days and weeks pass, the fire behind your burning desire could go out.

That's the beauty of harnessing the sexual force within you, because not only is it incredibly strong, but it's unlikely that your interest in sex is ever going to disappear. Now if you can fuse the sexual drive with another powerful emotion like love, you're really going to have an unstoppable force. That's why masturbation is so wildly popular and so constantly practiced. The key to it's popularity is that it fuses both those fine qualities in that it's sex with someone you love.

Curiously, this particular phenomena is even referred to in perhaps one of the most famous quotes in all of ancient Greek literature. When asked how the ancient Greek scholars got so much done with what little help they had, to a man they replied, "It is because the slave waits until the Master bates!"

The power of sex organs really is cosmic. It has been a topic of frequent discussion going back many thousands of years. Sex organs are tied in so inexorably with THE LIFEFORCE that you can't seperate them. Destroy one and you kill the other. The key question for you, at this point in the discussion, has to be, "How in the world does one tie their goals to their sex drives?" If you're not asking this question right now, you really should be!

The answer, which I know you're going to think sounds crazy, but I'm telling you it's crazy like a fox! The important thing here is that before I can tell you, you must promise not to talk about this or tell anyone you know! The reason is not what you might think. You're getting the final secret, after reading a well conceived and thoroughly researched compilation of important ideas, strung together like pearls on a necklace. For this reason, when I give you the final ingredient, you're getting a secret that makes your offensive game plan work with an extra measure of power that will virtually insure your skinniness!

This idea was first discussed by Napoleon Hill in his monumental best seller, "Think and Grow Rich." As the basis for the book, Hill studied the lives of ten of the most successful men in history, men who had risen to the very top of the age in which they lived. What Hill did was to isolate the qualities that all of these tremendously successful individuals had in common. The idea was to develop a path to success which all human beings could follow, simply by diligently and assiduously applying the learned qualities that each of these leaders took the time to acquire.

What Hill was able to demonstrate with his study was that there are clearly defined "success principles" common to all of the tremendously successful individuals he studied. Furthermore, he found that these principles were not inherent in these individuals from the beginning of their lives. They had to take the time and make the effort (often because life had dealt them such a miserable hand that they were forced) to go after these qualities with a laser beam like focus simply to survive.

You must attack your goal like [the classic story of] the lame child that wanted to learn to run so badly in order to play with his friends, that he practiced and practiced just to catch up and finally greatly surpassed them all. The crippled child, like many who start out way behind the eight ball and must strive like crazy just to catch up, often blow right past those who take what they have for granted and launch themselves to the very front of the pack because of their staunch determination to realize a burning goal held deep within.

Like a rubber band that's held back and finally allowed to fly, the power of an emotion filled desire, when unfrettered and allowed to hurl forward, will push individuals well beyond the crowd before they even think about stopping. What happens of course, is that in building up a huge reservoir of momentum, like a loaded freight train roaring down the track, they couldn't stop if they wanted to, and in point of fact, they usually don't. The fact that all of the men Hill studied had to overcome some handicap or disadvantage early in life is an indication that with a dream in your heart, a goal you must reach or parish in the attempt, there is absolutely no limit to what you can accomplish if you put your mind and soul into it! It has just been proven too many times, by people we wouldn't have given half a chance, not to believe it's true!

Hill wrote this book some sixty years ago, and it has become one of the most purchased books in the twentieth century. It has led innumerable people to success in their own lives and I think you'll find it interesting reading should you choose to do so. My point, however, is not in recommending the book as much as to highlight one of the qualities Hill found in all the people he studied. Hill referred to it as the transmutation of the sexual urge. But I can and will simplify it for you. Hill found, that without exception, each of the successful individuals he studied, took this river of strength (the sexual drive in each of us), and turned it just a little bit.

This turn was neither nasty or immoral or in any way evil, it was simply a channeling of the force. What each of these great individuals did that gave them such lasting consistency of purpose, was to fantasize about their goal so much that they began to get tremendous sexual gratification and great sexual pleasure from that which they wanted to accomplish!

To relate this to your goal of losing weight, when you are able to transmute your sexual desires to the point where losing weight will give you tremendous sexual pleasure, you will never need concern yourself with being fat again! When you eat your sex organs every day, combine your meals properly, drink all your water, and do daily aerobic exercises you will start to get thinner and thinner. But, you need to transmute and expand your sexual drives so that losing weight and getting to your goal brings you such tremendous, absolutely unbelievable, sexual pleasure that you never want to stop! Just stop and think for a moment how much weight you would actually lose, if losing that weight felt orgasmic! You'd be a stick!

As you do your visualizing and fantasizing about realizing your goal of losing weight and getting slim, you will want to tie this in with your sexual pleasure sense in a way that only you can manage. By expanding and developing this force within you, like the mighty rivers of the world that just keep coming, day after day, week after week, and year after year, you'll become relentless without having to try. Will power will be superfluous because the natural, but very powerful forces that you're about to harness will drive you. So that you don't have to force yourself to do what you know you should!

This transmutation of the sexual urge is alleged to be part of the success of top professionals in business and sports. They become so engrossed in their field of interest that consciously and unconsciously they begin finding tremendous sexual gratification in their work. They no longer look at work as a difficult, unbearable task but as something fun and enjoyable. Their work becomes their pleasure, and as a consequence, they just do it more. They think about it more and as a result, they can't wait to get back to it. In short, they love it. Their sexual drives have by no means become perverted, they've simply been channeled!

Conclusion

Losing weight may be a small goal for you, or it may be like taking on a second job, depending on how much you weigh now and what you intend to weigh at some point in the future. You can take losing excess weight just about as seriously as you want. What I've done for you is put together a plan that will, <u>every time,</u> lead you to the weight loss goal you crave. As we've mentioned, the beauty of the plan is that as you ramp up to D-DAY with your running start, your imagination and enthusiasm will induce you to make the effort needed to be successful. You will not need to force yourself to do a single thing!

The power of your mind is unparalleled as a force. Minds just like yours have created every device, built every bridge and building, and developed all the life giving medicines we have today. It is an absolute miracle of nature and you have one. Einstein estimated that we probably use less than 10% of our brain capacity. It has powers you've probably never used, but think of this. If Einstein is correct, and that by using the visualization and fantasy techniques you've been given, you're able to increase your total brain power by just 2%, you will have increased what you now use by 20%. Imagine a 20% increase in your brain power!

Einstein is said to have had a very vivid fantasy life and found great pleasure in it. Of course he didn't need to use visualization techniques to lose weight, but he did use them to solve troubling problems. In fact, he's an example of someone who started out behind the eight ball, having dyslexia and flunking the ninth grade the way he did. But when it came down to it, he channeled the forces within him to help him rewrite the laws of physics.

Believe me when I tell you that the list of great people who channeled and transmuted their sexual desires to achieve everything they ever had in mind is very long. Many of these people had to overcome hurdles a mile high. But they did it, and they did it by using their minds to produce from within themselves, a well spring of effort that enabled them to blow by the barricades standing before them.

The benefits of eating fruit in the morning are quite numerous and don't bear repeating here, as are the benefits of drinking plenty of water, properly combining your food and getting daily aerobic exercise, even if it's only a brisk walk. As you employ them, these keys will not fail you. Get your running start and go for it! Begin to visualize constantly. Don't neglect the Anal Power Technique, because there's something there you can harness. Fantasize about getting sexual pleasure from the weight loss process until the river of life flowing out of you builds such tremendous momentum that you become unstoppable!

As you start to fill yourself daily with THE LIFEFORCE and find that the extra energy you have improves and energizes you life, you won't be able to stop talking about it, it's that amazing. I would also ask you to drop me a line after you've tried it for a while and let me know how you're doing! I love success stories, and yours will be as important to you and, of course, to me, as Lincoln's, Einstein's, and so many others were to them and eventually to all the rest of us!

Thank you for buying the book and I hope with all my heart that you've found something that will help you to be permanently better! I know I have!

PREFACE TO APPENDIX SECTION

After reading the reviews of the first printing, I decided that I would incorporate some of the suggestions of the reviewers into appendixes which will serve to either add to existing information, clarify important points within the text, or simply make information available that was not enclosed within the body of the original text.

Some of the information contained in these appendixes is information or research which I had available when writing the book but chose not to include for fear of making the book too lengthy. After all, if you offer someone donuts, you don't necessarily want to give them the whole tray, even if they CAN eat them all.

In addition, based on people's reading habits, thicker books tend to lessen the chance that they will be grabbed up off the shelf, and if you don't read it, what good is it? With that in mind, I decided that it would be much quicker and easier to get the new and often requested information into your hands by way of a simple appendix section, rather than try to weave it into the text and take a chance on interrupting the smooth flow I've worked so hard to achieve.

Even though you have reached the official conclusion, I hope you will choose to read the appendixes and use them to supplement and reinforce what you've just read. I say this because I myself know full well how easy it is to blow off reading appendixes. But as I've said, I wrote them because people just like you requested the information, and I hope you enjoy them. If there is any further information in connection with the diet you'd like to see in print, please don't hesitate to write and let me know!

JOHN VAN REGINALD TOMLINSON III

APPENDIX 1
- A LIST OF VARIOUS SEX ORGANS

The first thing that comes to mind when compiling a list of sex organs is that you've probably already learned to identify sex organs on sight. Furthermore, you no doubt have already decided which sex organs you like the best. If that's the case, I encourage you to eat 'em to your heart's content. The important thing, once again, is to eat them raw! I cannot stress this enough. This way you get THE LIFEFORCE as well as the pleasure, the water, the soluble fiber, and the fructose.

I should mention at this point, that while I haven't given as much attention to vegetables, they're obviously essential to your diet because of the many good things they contain. So when you eat them, as eat them you must, make sure that they are fresh or fresh frozen as well. Vegetables, as you might have guessed, contain THE LIFEFORCE. But because they aren't directly responsible for the propagation of their kind, it may not be as strong. So getting them out of a can should be your last source of choice. When they're canned, they're cooked to death (the same goes for fruit) before you ever get your hands on them. So that even if you don't re-cook them before eating them, very little of their health giving properties remain.

Now back to fruits. The first thing that makes a fruit easy to detect is that, being a reproductive organ, it will, if planted (unless of course, it's a hybrid), produce another of its species. This means that it's either a seed or contains the seeds inside its casing (as in high water content fruits) which enable the plant to reproduce. I'm telling you this now because the following list of sex organs is not meant to be an exhaustive, all encompassing list of all the sex organs found on earth. In fact, I'm quite sure there are a number of sex organs that I've never seen or even heard about, although I'm sure I'd like to. If you run into some that you think I'd enjoy, send a picture so that I can see what they look like, and I'll keep an eye pealed for them (whatever that means).

I'll list them alphabetically and avoid listing all the various types within the species, as in the case of apples, among others, where it isn't important to do so.

APPLES
APRICOTS
BANANAS
BERRIES: black & red rasp, black, blue, boysen,
              mul, and strawberries.

CHERRIES   MANGO
CURRENTS   MELONS: (these are my favorite
GRAPEFRUIT   for breakfast!)
GRAPES   NECTARINES
GUAVAS   ORANGES
KIWI   PAPAYA

PEACHES   POMEGRANATES
PEARS   TANGELOS
PERSIMMONS   TANGERINES
PINEAPPLES   UGLY FRUIT
PLUMS

The next list is comprised of fruits that are generally referred to as vegetables but are by definition fruits. These fruits aren't generally as high in water content, and as a result become of secondary importance during breakfast. But they are sex organs and do contain THE LIFEFORCE.

CUCUMBER
EGGPLANT
GRAINS: oats, wheat, rye, barley, bulgur, and unprocessed   rice, and corn.
GREEN BEANS
LEGUMES: black-eyed peas, chickpeas, great north ern beans, kidney beans, lentils, lima beans, navy beans, peanuts, pinto beans, soy beans, and split peas.
NUTS & SEEDS: (these should be avoided like all fruits when cooked, roasted or salted!)
PEAS: (with or without pods)
PEPPERS
SQUASH: everything from acorn to zucchini
TOMATOES

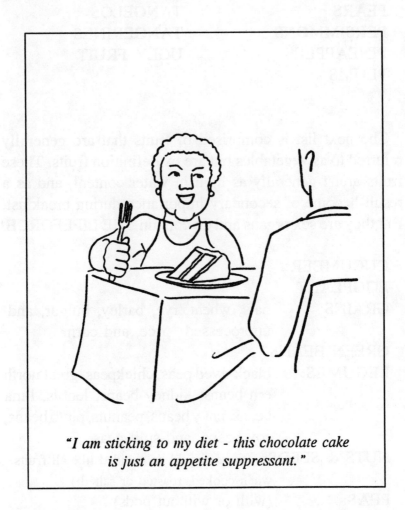

"I am sticking to my diet - this chocolate cake
is just an appetite suppressant."

APPENDIX 2
- HUNGER

There's an old Scottish line that goes, "They always talk about my drinking, but they never talk about my thirst." The same can be said for most diets, in that they're always talking to you about how much you can eat, but they don't seem to talk much about your hunger. Therefore, this appendix will do just that. We need to take a closer look at the concept of "Just In Time Inventories" and how it breaks the cycle of starving and binge eating that so many dieters seem to fall into.

You may remember early in the book we talked about the elaborate safeguard system the body has against starvation by, among other things, dramatically reducing the number of calories it burns for energy by reducing thyroid output, when it senses that its intake has been curtailed. In fact, the body has a system to safeguard itself against many threats and dangers that might bring injury, starvation is only one example. That's why the body produces so many different feelings, many of which are created solely for the purpose of prompting you to an action of some sort. Fear is another classic example of this process because it motivates you to safeguard the system by reducing the threat in some way, whether it's to run, fight or in some way eliminate the problem entirely. Even the pleasure of sex is designed as a motivator to help continue the species.

In short, the body causes you to act in ways that attempt to assure its self-preservation. To be sure, the body will do its part to aid you in developing an action plan to increase your safety. In the case of fear, the body has a small gland on the kidney produce adrenalin, which makes both your mind and your muscles work with greater efficiency. The preservation instinct is so strong that the mind is CON-STANTLY looking for danger. It takes in new data moment by moment and compares it with the known outcomes from previous circumstances. This is called anticipation. As it anticipates, it begins to implement preventive and corrective strategies to minimize the possibility of the danger actually transpiring.

Hunger is one of the body's many warning signals. It's the body's way of telling you that your blood sugar level is getting low. It's like the oil light coming on in your car. A message is being sent by your engine, asking you to do something to prevent a problem. You can certainly ignore the message, but you run a risk. Listening to your body is even more important that listening to your car engine, because when you don't listen to your body it makes your life miserable until you do.

"Just In Time Inventories" means having just enough of whatever it is you're storing to finish the job. The advantage of using this type of storage system is that when your body begins to realize that food will always be on the way shortly, it loses the need to store fat for protection against a future period of famine. The net effect of using this type of storage system is that the brain (which as you may remember has incredible control over each cell in your body) will realize that if the needed supplies are always going to arrive on time, it has way too much inventory stored for an event that now appears unlikely. This realization prompts the brain to begin, slowly at first, to eliminate excess fat from the body. Furthermore, it will make less fat in the future and will actively work to keep you in a reduced inventory situation as long as you continue to be just in time!

The problem you've got, particularly if you've been on reduced calorie diets intermittently in the past, is that it's going to take a while for your body to believe in your ability to be reliable. Your genetic code retains instincts learned from your ancient ancestors. These instinctual body functions go back to when people needed to store a great deal of fat to protect themselves against the irregularity of meals and the coming winter. When you try to starve yourself skinny, these bodily processes, which are as old as father time and mother nature, will foil your every attempt!

This is why people go from what the body perceives as famine everytime they try to starve themselves skinny, to ravaging hunger, which precipatates another binge. What happens is that when you start eating again, your body immediately begins to protect you against the next period of starvation. It makes and stores extra fat, because fat is, ounce for ounce, the most efficient store of energy it has. To illustrate what I mean, the store of energy in one gram of protein is four calories, one gram of carbohydrate also has four calories, but one gram of fat has nine calories. One gram of fat will produce more than twice the energy of either carbohydrates or proteins. With that in mind, it should be easy to understand why the body stores fat. If it stored anything else we'd be many times bigger than we are!

Another interesting thing about the body is that the minute you go off a reduced calorie diet, your body will induce you to eat that which is most readily turned into fat. It will build the protection it thinks it needs into your system as quickly as possible because it has no idea how soon the next famine will start and it has be ready. But simply having your body put the fat back isn't the worst of the damage you do when you try to starve yourself thin.

Let me illustrate what I mean. Lets say you starve yourself until you lose twenty pounds. Of that twenty pounds, five will be water, five will be fat, and ten will be muscle. The Body will sense that reduction, get paranoid about starving and in order to make sure that it will continue to have plenty of fat to burn (fat is utilized for about 2/3 of the body's energy production), the body will increase it's fat producing enzyme, Lipase, by as much as ten times the normal amount found in the body. From the time the "famine" period ends it can take as long as eighteen weeks for lipase to return to normal levels.

Furthermore, the reason you lose muscle is that it's a ready source of protein. Protein, as mentioned earlier in the book, can be converted to sugar through the process known as gluconeogensis. When the brain needs sugar and can't get it orally, the muscles are the FIRST to go! Because unfortunately for us, once sugar is turned to fat with Lipase, it can't be turned back again. If the body can't get you to eat something it can convert to sugar (primarily carbohydrates), it'll start liquidating your muscles. Due to the fact that the brain and body have to have sugar to operate (the body needs sugar for a huge number of various processes, not the least of which is burning fat), when you try to starve yourself thin, you will dissolve your muscles in the process.

When you revert back to your previous level of intake, which is almost certain to happen (because of their artificial nature, reduced calorie diets are impossible to sustain), your body accelerates the fat building process, as we just mentioned. But in addition to that, you've now got an even bigger problem, because when the twenty pounds go back on, as they inevitably do, you'll put on five pounds of water and fifteen pounds of fat, leaving the ten pounds of muscle somewhere in the dust.

What this means to you is that, on top of the fact that you'll now be weaker and tire more easily as a result of having less muscle, the muscle itself burns 50 calories per pound per day, so in essence you've just gotten rid of the very thing in your body that burns fat for you, muscle! This means that once you gain the twenty pounds back, it'll be even harder to stay at that weight level from that point forward. Your body is going to burn fewer calories every day until you replace the muscle you lost. If you don't replace the muscle with exercise, you'll probably gain more than the original twenty back! That's why reduced calorie diets MUST be accompanied by aerobic exercise to even have a snowball's chance of working.

This is why people who diet the most usually weigh the most. Just like you can't beat the casinos in Las Vegas, even though you might get ahead temporarily, you can't beat your body at a game it knows far better than you do. You must realize that the game is rigged right from the start. Your body has the ability to create feelings like hunger whenever it wants and you have to suffer through them, almost without end sometimes.

Simply put, your body will always be able to force your hand by using your feelings against you! So if you don't get in harmony with your body first, your chance of permanently shedding weight is about as good as my chance of having kids. If you doubt the strength of these bodily instincts from long ago, do a little experiment which will prove beyond all doubt just how enduring they are. Take a kitten from its mother just after birth. This way it will be impossible for it to learn any cat habits from its Mommy. Naturally you'll have to feed it to keep it alive, but that's understood. What you will find, as a result of this experiment is that as the kitten grows, not only will it be a pain in the butt, but it will manifest all the cat habits of it's ancestors, without learning any of them from you or another cat.

Your body has the very same instinctual memory and just as you can't keep a kitten from licking it's paws, you can't stop your body from piling up fat if you send it the wrong signals. This is why THE FABULOUS SEX ORGAN DIET is so perfect for permanent weight loss, because it allows you to eat something whenever you're hungry. Just In Time means just in time, and in order for your body to believe that you truly want to employ this system, you must answer the call when you get hungry with something good. Whether you drink a big glass of water to stir up the partially digested food in the intestines, eat a piece of fruit, have a salad or a plate of pasta, you must never let your hunger become pronounced!

There are only two ways to break the starvation and binge cycle. You can fast until you get anorexia, or eat normally. I have found eating normally to be the best choice. Either you starve so long that it becomes a permanent condition, or you keep your body so well supplied that it loses sight of the starvation threat and stops piling up fat. Obviously, well supplied in this case refers to quality not quantity. You should always adhere to the basic tenants of THE FABULOUS SEX ORGAN DIET, which means eating as much fruit as you can possibly eat in the morning and never mixing heavy foods with starches the rest of the day.

This naturally gives rise to the question of cravings, which seem to be the bane of dieters everywhere. I have only two things to say about cravings. First, all humans have, in their control center, an exact idea of how much intake is needed to refuel. Babies and little children start out on the "Just In Time" inventory control system. They eat when they're hungry. They won't eat when they're not hungry. They eat until they're full and then they won't eat another bite. Kids that are allowed to eat when they get hungry and aren't forced to eat when they're not, won't get fat! Kids only get fat when they're forced to eat more than they want or when they try to control their weight by reducing their intake, and thus putting themselves on the fat accumulation cycle.

Kids and animals are very tuned in to their fuel needs. You can leave the tastiest food imaginable out for a pet but when they're done, they just won't eat. They have no compunction to clean up their bowl! When they're done, they're done. They listen to their bodies and since their bodies don't have to fear starvation, they don't get fat. It should be noted however, that pets can learn poor dietary habits living with humans and actually get fat in the process. This is primarily the result of either not being allowed to get out and run or living with neurotic adults.

Animals in the wild never get fat.

Another reason dieters sometimes gorge themselves on such things as cakes, cookies and pies is that they're deriving a secret pleasure from doing something they perceive as naughty. Tremendous pleasure can be had from doing that which we sense we shouldn't be doing. This is one of the peculiarities in man's nature. In fact the phenomena is so wide spread, that eating goodies we shouldn't is only one small example. We see this secret pleasure sense in everything from kids who swipe a watermelon from the farmers melon patch to get a much better tasting watermelon than the one they could buy at the store; to the excitement young people find in doing naughty things like pre-marital sex. An example of this phenomena seen over and over again, is the individual who is quite sexually active while single, but once married and sex is suddenly quite permissible, they lose all interest in it, much to the dismay of their partner.

It's human nature to want what we don't think we can have. Whether it's sex or potato chips the principle is the same. Fortunately the cure is relatively simple in the case of sugar laden starches. Just realize that you can have all you want, any time you want and there is nobody stopping you. How much of this stuff would you want, if somebody sat you down every day and forced you to eat things like cakes and pies? You'd soon lose interest, because like most people, you don't like things that are forced on you.

The point is, since you're now in command, you get to make the decisions. You're in charge of the way you look and the way you feel. You get to make your own rules! If you want to go out every day and eat three or four cakes, a couple of pies and a few dozen cookies, do it! It's completely all right for point proving purposes, and it can certainly all be squeezed into the dietary regimen I'm proposing.

The first thing that happens when you realize, possibly for the first time in your life, that eating all you want (especially when it comes to sex organs), isn't naughty, is that you either go out and satiate your repressed desire for goodies until you just can't lift another cake or you lose interest altogether. In either case, once you realize that you can eat anything you want, your wants start to come into line with your body's needs. You begin to eat until you're full of it and then you stop. You quit trying to put twenty gallons of fuel into an eighteen gallon tank. If you eat all the foods you're supposed to eat, you aren't going to have room for junk. But you can have it if you want it. My guess is that you just won't want it.

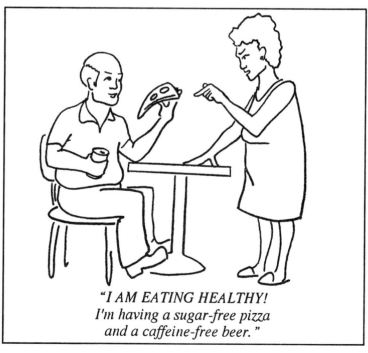

"I AM EATING HEALTHY!
I'm having a sugar-free pizza
and a caffeine-free beer."

The idea behind "Just In Time" inventory control is cosmic because it takes all the stress out of eating. You start eating to live rather than living to eat. That's the way you were as a child, before the world got a hold on you, and that's the way you can be again. This also highlights the stupidity of diet foods. If you're going to convince your body not to carry excess inventory, you can't be filling up on foods with no fuel value. It might fool your tastebuds going down, but it isn't going to fool your body when it tries to burn the stuff because there's nothing there to burn.

Eating diet food is like getting your car ready for a long trip by filling the tank with water, the needle will certainly read full but your engine knows better. Don't cheat your body! You are in charge of what you eat and you can eat whatever and whenever you want. Just be smart! Diet food won't sustain life, it only serves to promote a deception, while your body continues to get hungry. Obviously reducing fat intake can make some sense if you are trying to lose fat. But if you cut all the fat out of your diet and increase your carbohydrate intake as a result, your body can still turn around and make literally as much fat as it wants, if it perceives a lack of balance, and what have you really gained?

The point is that once you realize that you're in charge of your eating habits and can do anything you damned well please in this free country of ours, you'll do things because they make sense, not because there's a secret pleasure attached. Now granted, even though you're free to eat cake after cake if you so desire (and if you've got to do it to prove to yourself that you are indeed free, don't hesitate), you've got to remember that freedom has a price, and that price is responsibility.

Money is a pretty common want in our society and we all know that the banks and the bankers are full of it most of the time. I myself generally want more money than I have and you probably could use a little more yourself. Now you and I are both basically free to walk into any bank any day of the week and rob it. But we don't, because we know we'll have to take responsibility for that act sooner or later. We have therefore decided, of our own free will, that we won't rob banks because we don't want to suffer the ultimate consequence, even though initially you could probably get all the money you could carry.

As a result of this decision, you can drive by banks all day long and not feel compelled to take their money. While you'd love to have the money, you don't care for the repercussions that would result from acting in a manner that isn't best. It's a classic example of making a rational decision based on a SEPARATION OF OUR WANTS and you can do the very same thing with food and eating.

Once you're on THE FABULOUS SEX ORGAN DIET for a while and you've eaten plenty of good food (getting full but not stuffed meal after meal), you'll make the same sort of decisions about food and eating, as you do about bank robbery. It's all based on your own personal separation of wants. Once you become relentless in the pursuit of a lighter body and are able to get off the starvation and binge cycle so common to dieters (by eating good food regularly), you will definitely be able to broaden your separation of wants beyond a simple lack of interest in robbing banks and realize that you can do the same thing for cakes, pies, cookies, donuts and a whole list of things the body craves when it must make fat. This is part of the healing process!

Remember, the body craves those things which produce fat the quickest, because it has a built in system which demands it. If you try to fight it by doing something artificial and completely unsustainable, your subsequent hunger, and the volume of consumption it promotes, will amaze friend and foe alike. But if you work with your system by eating well whenever you're hunger alarm goes off (keeping in mind of course, just what eating well is, based on our previous discussions), you'll be able to walk by a nice looking cake and not want to eat it for the very same reason you go by banks and don't feel like robbing them.

On THE FABULOUS SEX ORGAN DIET you will lose interest in doing the wrong thing and gain interest in doing the right thing as you put starvation and binges behind you.

Conclusion

Remember, in going to "Just In Time" inventory control, it is extremely counterproductive to let yourself get overly hungry for any reason and particularly for weight loss purposes! For your body to trust you, you have to begin to trust your body and eat WHEN it asks you to, but not necessarily WHAT it asks you to. Just In Time means just in time. If you'll do this, you'll convince your body that there is no need to store vast reserves for the future. As you do this, that marvelous control mechanism you possess, will start making you skinny!

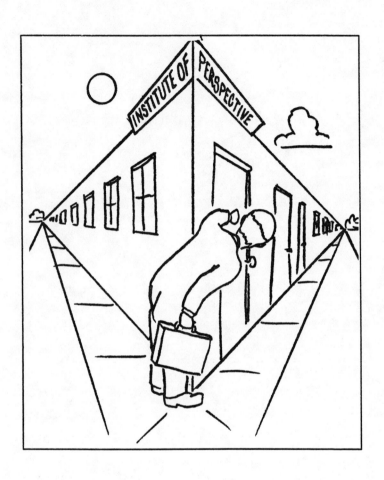

APPENDIX 3
- THE RELATIONSHIP BETWEEN TIME AND RESULTS

Ben Franklin was the first guy to say that time is money. Unfortunately, you can't measure time in days the way you can measure money in dollars because every day is different. We talk about having good days and bad days, but we rarely talk about having good dollars or bad dollars. But no matter, whether it's days or dollars, or just dollar days, what we should be talking about, is that regardless of their merits, amounts of both are relative.

Think about it. You could make the statement, "Gee, that took a hell of a long time." And in the very next breath you could say, "Boy, that was really quick." If, in the first statement, you're talking about waiting a half an hour to get a fast food burger, you'd be correct by all standards of decency. Yet, if the second statement referred to the fact that it only took one week for your bank to enable you to close on a house, you'd probably be talking about banks on Mars.

The point is, that regardless of how much time something takes, it's only long or short in relation to some other event, not to itself. This is a key concept to keep in mind, because whether it takes three weeks or three months to lose the weight you want to lose, the benefits are simply too enormous to ignore. But you should never compare your progress in the weight loss arena to ordering burgers, because your goal is permanent weight loss, not a quick, sharp drop in your tonnage.

Think of it this way, if you cut yourself, the length of time it takes to heal depends on a multitude of factors, including but not limited to: how deep it is, how fast your body can corral the necessary resources to start rebuilding, where it's located on the body (is it a high use area?), is there infection present, or even if it was closed up with stitches. When you're overweight, your body has a repair job to do. Even if you want it to heal as fast as humanly possible, you must endure a chain of events transpiring within your body over which you possess only limited control. Fortunately, this limited control is the margin of difference between whether it happens or it doesn't.

Remember, you're still the one that decides, you just shouldn't expect to bake a cake from scratch in ten minutes!

These words are not meant to in any way impede you in your relentless quest for destiny, they are only meant to add perspective and to prevent discouragement from derailing you before you get across the river. Consider this, when you begin this dietary regimen and activity enhanced program, you're starting in motion numerous chemical changes in your body that accelerate the fat burning process. Once these are in place, your body will burn five to six hundred more calories every day than it did previously. However, because this process is somewhat dependent on a bodily increase in the production of certain enzymes, you will be burning many more calories three months into the diet than you will be on the first day, even if you do exactly the same thing on both days.

The same thing can be said for the habits you alter. Your habits will make you more or less efficient as a human being, depending upon how closely correlated they are to your chosen goals. As you employ all the habit altering techniques we discussed such as the running start, visualization, never skipping meals, using Just In Time inventories for energy production and becoming relentless, your body will obviously be more tuned in to you and you to your body. For these reasons, three months into the program, life will be much better for you than on the very first day, even if you do more the first day than the ninetieth day.

Breaking the body's fear of starvation alone, especially if you've been on numerous reduced calorie diets, is going to take some time. But like the tiny snowball rolling down the long hill, the whole process continues to accelerate as your internal health improves! When you act in a certain way, your body will act in a certain way in response, of this you can be absolutely certain. If you care for a deep cut, it will heal. If you rub dirt in it every day, it won't, and in fact will probably only get worse. But no matter how much you care for it, it's still going to heal at it's own rate. Your contentment comes in the knowledge that if you continue to care for it, it will heal!

For this reason, weighing yourself is of only secondary importance. When you weigh in, you can only get one of three readings: higher than the last reading, the same, or lower. Two out of the three have the potential for producing some level of disappointment. So you've got a

67% chance of being discouraged before you start, and it's almost a certainty that you're not getting the whole story, no matter what the number. What you should expect is that permanent weight loss is best achieved at a rate of 1% to 1.5% of your total body weight per week. In other words, at 200 pounds you should expect to permanently lose 2 to 3 pounds per week. The thing is, it isn't a straight line effect. It might be down four pounds one week, and up two the next, or it might be up a pound and then down four.

Here's why. Everyone's body goes through a monthly cycle, the woman's being the more obvious of the two, but regardless of your sex, your weight will vary over the course of the cycle. If you happen to catch a wave while weighing yourself, it's of little consequence to the over all process, because weight loss is, in its essence, chemistry, and chemical reactions are incredibly consistent. If they weren't, life as we know it could not exist. The fat burning process going on in your body is every bit as reliable as the reaction you get when you mix vinegar and baking soda. The speed of the reaction is the only variable.

That's why time is not nearly as important as you think. Your body is like a great big test tube, and if you mix in all the ingredients, weight loss has to occur! But the process will inevitably change speeds depending on such things as temporary increases and decreases in fat burning efficiency. That's why you'll have a plateau from time to time. But they normally last only one to two weeks and then the process resumes. Knowing this will take the focus off the time frame and put it squarely on improving your health.

But if you must weigh yourself, you're better off weighing yourself every single day, keeping a written record and charting the weekly average (the average is found by adding all seven numbers and dividing by seven). This way you'll become intimately familiar with your monthly cycles and the reading you get on any one particular day will be almost meaningless. This way you'll clearly see the trend, which of course, is all that's really important for permanent weight loss.

Finally, while it's easy to see why time is money in the business world, in the weight loss world, time heals all wounds, but money cannot. Money can't buy you good health, but if you do the right things, time will lay it at your feet! Think of it this way, at five years of age, a year seems like an eternity, because even one of 'em is a big percentage of your entire life. A five year old really hasn't seen that many of them go by and at best, is uncertain what's coming next. At sixty, a year is a much smaller frame of reference. In percentage terms, for the person at sixty, one year is the equivalent of six days to the five year old.

Yes, time is relative. If you're thirty, look back at how long you've been here on the planet and realize that if you're healthy, the odds are that you've got more than twice that length of time left to go. If you're forty and healthy, as long as you've lived, and as many things as you've done, you've got that much more time left to go. When you think in these terms, what is an allocation of three to six months in order to make the next fifty years bounding with vivacious energy? Instead of continuing down the same path and becoming progressively more sluglike. Choose health, but don't be held hostage to time in the meantime!

Conclusion

Remember, even a 1% change will make a huge difference in where you end up over time. If Saddam Hussein had the ability to make only a 1% change in the course in his scud missiles, they would have all hit vital areas, instead of falling harmlessly in the desert or at sea, the way that most, but not all of the missiles that were fired, did. So please don't minimize even a 1% change, in your daily behavior. Making small regular changes, like changing the degree heading on a compass, can mean the difference between getting to where you're going and remaining hopelessly adrift.

The important thing is to gain perspective and be patient with yourself and your body. If you follow THE FABULOUS SEX ORGAN DIET you will become permanently thin. It doesn't take money, it only takes time.

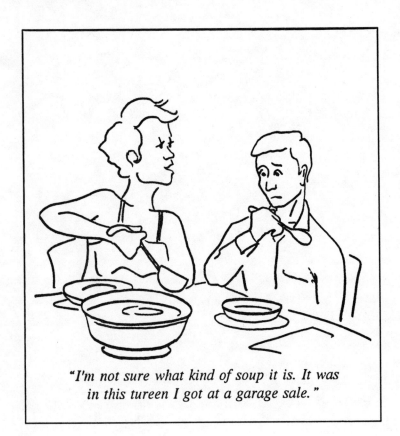

"I'm not sure what kind of soup it is. It was in this tureen I got at a garage sale."

APPENDIX 4
- MEAL IDEAS

From the beginning, I have been opposed to filling the book with such things as charts, recipes, and a daily dietary regimen for two reasons: 1) Some of the people who write diet books for a living do that kind of thing to make a very thin book look fat, and I wanted to give you more than your money's worth, not less. 2) The whole idea behind the success of this diet is that there is no artificial structure that you must adhere to for some fixed period of time in order to lose weight. Once you understand the ancient dietary principles that foster good health, the daily dietary regimen you adhere to will be completely unique to you. Your daily dietary regimen should be something that not only keeps you healthy but serves your needs and wants, not mine or anybody else's.

All volume measurements you see on strict diets are based on statistical averages. I believe that once you know the story, you'll be the best judge of how much is right for you. As long as you eat until you're full, but not jam packed, you'll be fine. All human beings, except for maybe the Germans and the Japs, rebel at fixed, rigid structures, no matter what they're for. It's one of the two reasons why people fail when dieting. It's almost impossible for the average person to stick to something artificial in nature for very long, regardless of its degree of difficulty.

THE FABULOUS SEX ORGAN DIET lets you be the judge every day. As a consequence of this, it is very easy to make this dietary regimen a permanent part of the way you live. Once the principles are so ingrained within that you don't have to think about what to eat, or even how to eat, you'll get skinny and stay skinny long after you've forgotten where this damned book is. I want you to keep re-reading this book to pick up new ideas, not because you have to be reminded what to eat.

With that said, I have decided to make a small concession to my beloved editors and detail what I might eat on an average day. This is only a snapshot however, and it is not my intention to in any way impose a meal structure on you, but you show you how it works.

BREAKFAST

FRUIT JUICE - fresh or fresh frozen. Drink it with your vitamin. I use Theragram M because each capsule contains not only vitamins but minerals important to the fat burning process. I probably wouldn't hesitate to use a generic copy.

FRUIT: several slices of Honey Dew melon a couple of slices of Cantaloupe 1 or 2 slices of Watermelon 5 to 10 strawberries and maybe a small bunch of seedless grapes

NOTE: my wife cuts the melon off the rind and into bite sized chunks for ease of consumption, bless her heart.

BIG GLASS OF WATER This is a great time to knock off some of those daily ounces. Have a few more glasses before lunch.

LUNCH: Remember this is where you start to properly combine your meals. Have either meat or starch as the main dish, but never both!

SOUP: If I'm having some sort of meat as the main course I'll have vegetable soup -- no crackers. Don't eat gravy based soups or stews with meat meals because the gravy is made with starch. If the soup is great, I will often just have a couple of bowls and maybe some salad for lunch.

SALAD: It's always good. If you tried to get your total daily caloric need from lettuce you'd have to eat 40 pounds. Unless you're having a starch meal, avoid croutons. Avoid bacon bits all together.

MAIN ENTREE: Grilled breast of chicken or a grilled piece of fish. Avoid breading and sauces because of their starch nature. All spices are fine.

VEGGIES: Steamed or microwaved is best. Avoid anything out of an institutional sized can, or any can for that matter. Avoid cream sauces.

DESSERT: This is at your discretion. If you're stuffed already, avoid becoming a compactor. I find that generally, but not always, a couple of tastes to get the flavor in my mouth is just as satisfying as eating the entire dessert.

NOTE: Sandwiches are only permitted if they're vegetarian in nature because you shouldn't eat a meat and a starch together. Of course, if you can make the sandwich with a non starch casing...

SNACKS: Healthy snacks are healthy and I encourage them if you need to refuel. Don't drive your body until the tank is completely dry, ever! The first thing to do whenever you get in the mood to snack is to drink a big glass of water to stir up the food that's already down there. If you want more, have some fruit, a salad, a cup of soup or a vegetarian sandwich. A healthy snack about 4:00 p.m. to 4:30 p.m. is a great way to ruin your appetite or allow you to push dinner back to the 6:00 to 7:00 p.m. area, whichever is more convenient for you. Having dinner later will reduce any possible interest in a late night snack.

SUPPER: This meal is interchangeable with lunch as far as what's available. It should be lighter than lunch if possible.

DINNER
SALAD: Big salads with pieces of barbecued chicken are great, as an entire meal particularly in

the summer, during hot weather. Something like this is often all you want.

ENTREE: I love pasta meals here. This is a great time for an all starch meal. You can do a million things with pasta, vegetables, and sauces. You might also try partially cooking potatoes, allowing them to remain somewhat crunchy with the skin on. In this state, potatoes are a huge source of vitamin C among other things. A potato is much more enjoyable if you don't cook it to death. Try 'em this way with ketchup, or sour cream, they're great!

DESSERT: You're wide open. If you've eaten plenty of good food, you're entitled. Just make sure you've eaten plenty of good food first! Remember the dessert is the frosting on the cake of a fine meal, too much frosting on a cake...

LATE NIGHT: Obviously this is the least best time to eat,
SNACKS but sometimes you just have to. My feeling is that if your body says you really have to, you should listen. The first best thing to do is drink a big glass of water. The second best thing to do is to eat something good before you eat something not so good. The third best thing to do is work on improving your dietary behavior with the ANAL POWER TECHNIQUE!

That's the whole enchilada. Once you get the hang of eating this way, you'll thin down to where you want to be without feeling in any way put out. If you continue to eat in the above specified manner once you've hit your goal and continue to take daily exercise, you'll not only stay thin for the rest of the many remaining years of your life, but you'll CONTINUE to feel happier and more energetic than ever. What more can one ask?

Before I let you go on to the next appendix, I want to briefly discuss two things in conjunction with eating. The first concerns drinking alcohol and smoking pot. They both have demonstrated the ability to dramatically lower one's resolve in the face of food. When you eat under the influence of either of these two drugs, you are almost, by definition, out of control. This can lead to eating a tremendous volume of food long after you're no longer hungry. Obviously this isn't a good idea, so be very careful, because they both make weight loss much more of a job!

In addition, drinking alcohol can be compared to pouring raw sugar down your throat. It sounds fun, but it's not. It's just more to metabolize. Further, pot screws up your blood sugar sensor, which can lead to a hunger that knows no bounds. So be careful that your lust for pleasure doesn't give your new and improved dietary regimen a flat tire. Use them only for medicinal purposes.

The second thing I want to discuss is your metabolism. The metabolism is simply the sum total of the body's energy usage. Whatever the process, if it involves energy utilization, it's part of your metabolism. Your body's single biggest source of energy is fat. When you increase your metabolism you increase fat usage. Since muscle movement, especially sustained muscle movement, has the biggest single effect on the level of metabolism in your body, the more you use your muscles, the more you'll burn fat.

Furthermore, the longer the muscle, the more it stimulates the metabolism. Leg and buttocks muscles have the potential to burn the most, not only because they are the longest muscles in the body, but because they haul a lot of weight around with every step. For this reason, walking will burn as many calories as running, provided you walk the same distance you would have run. So if you're really over weight, don't run, walk! Your joints will thank you and you'll still enjoy the benefits of an elevated metabolism.

In addition, while it is not widely known, eating itself raises the metabolism of the body significantly. The reason should be obvious to you after reading this book. Eating uses so many different muscles in the body, that when they're all activated, along with your glands, the metabolic rate goes up. Exercising, when your metabolic rate is already elevated, provides a slingshot effect, when it comes to the body's ability to metabolize fat. Therefore, it should be clear to you that the very best time to walk or exercise is either before or after a meal.

Your body's metabolic rate is at its low ebb just moments before you wake in the morning. This is referred to as your basil or base rate. From the moment you wake, it starts to rise, and peaks somewhere between 4:00 to 8:00 p.m. After which it begins to wind down until it hits its low ebb again the next morning. In effect, your metabolism ebbs and flows like the tide, and catching high tide to work out makes sailing out of the harbor much easier if you're a big boat!

Exercising will not only elevate your metabolism while you work out, but it will stay at a higher than normal rate for the remainder of the time you are awake. There is often even a residual effect that carries into the next day, especially if you're in shape. Thus, over time, daily exercise is very desirable because it serves to permanently increase the daily caloric utilization of your metabolism by five to six hundred calories. This is enough to keep you forever skinny, providing you do things as simple as eating right and take daily walks or exercise before or after meals!

APPENDIX 5
- DAIRY PRODUCTS

I am often asked, "What about dairy products?" My response is often, "What about 'em?" They're fun, they're tasty, and they are, along with meat, the biggest source of saturated fat and cholesterol available today. How can you say no to that?

Milk is 3.5% protein, 3.5% fat, 4.9% carbohydrate, and 87% water by volume. Under any circumstances, drinking milk is better than drinking pop, especially with cookies, fudge brownies, or virtually anything chocolate, because it has the subtle effect of creating nutritional content in the snack. It's also a better drink than coffee and can be great for mid-afternoon refueling. The only problem is that for many people it's difficult to digest. That's why cows don't even drink it.

The worse culprits however, would have to be considered hard cheeses and ice cream. If you can find it in your heart to say good-bye to these surly sources of fat, your heart will thank you. Saturated fat, which as you remember from our earlier discussions, is the type of fat found in the skillet after you cook a burger. It hardens at room temperature. The old time thinking by dietary scientists was that (because of the protein found in cheese), even if you were now too old to cut the mustard, you were never too old to cut the cheese.

But as you might have guessed, thanks to the EPA this thinking has changed. The current estimate is that about 97% of the fat you eat remains fat, if it is in fact taken up by your system. That's why we're witnessing the current bandwagon in the scientific community to avoid anything with fat in it. They reason that if you start out by eating less fat, you'll be skinnier. It sounds good but it isn't necessarily true, because your system is far more complex than that. Balance is usually both the problem and the solution!

The bottom line on this nut shell, without rehashing the science involved, is that THE FABULOUS SEX ORGAN DIET strives for complete and utter balance within your system. A little of this or a little of that once your system is in balance is virtually immaterial. Take eggs for example, they're a great source of protein, but the yoke's a tremendous source of cholesterol. Due to the fact that the protein is available from other sources many dietary scientists recommend avoiding them altogether in order to avoid the cholesterol. But most of the cholesterol in your body doesn't come from eating cholesterol, it comes from available fat in the system.

The point is, if cholesterol is backing up in your system it's because other things are out of balance, not because you happen to eat an egg now and again. Things usually back up in the system when there's a problem somewhere. If, as an example, it was determined that you have way too much ammonia in your system, a diagnostician won't tell you to drink less ammonia, they'll look into why it isn't being processed correctly. Doctors often don't have the slightest as to why someone's cholesterol is backing up, but generally speaking, it's because there is a lack of balance somewhere in the system.

For that reason, I'm not going to sit here today and tell you not to eat the mounds of fat found in dairy products because if you're living according to THE FABULOUS SEX ORGAN DIET it's immaterial. You're never going to have a chance to eat mounds of fat on this dietary regimen because there's already so much to eat, you're going to be hard pressed to find time eat everything you already have before you! As an example, when would you have time to eat eggs and sausages if you first eat tons of fruit until noon?

The true beauty of THE FABULOUS SEX ORGAN DIET is that you're doing so much, in terms of both quality AND quantity to restore the natural bodily harmony within you, that you never get to those things that promote disharmony. The choices are always yours, and as you continue to choose health, you'll find that a number of foods will become irrelevant!

THE EPILOGUE
- PERSISTENCE
AND PERSEVERANCE

I have learned a lesson from the rushing waters of a mountain stream, and that is that there are no insurmountable obstacles. Fore, the steady pressure against the rock by the water always wins out in the end.

It shows me the power in never giving up, in never quitting. Fore, no rock, not even the hardest of rocks, is immune to power of a rushing stream.

Is it not the persevering soul, the one who conquers or dies, the one who shall win in the end, because he has worn down the resistance to the point of its collapse, by pushing on until he finally reached the sea of his joy?

For a river to stagnate must certainly mean its death. But when it continues to push ahead, and by doing so remain in life's flow, it will be fed along its' way by unseen springs and streams so as to nourish it in its pursuit of destiny.

JOHN VAN REGINALD TOMLINSON III

Notes: